LINKING MIGRATION, HIV/AIDS AND URBAN FOOD SECURITY IN SOUTHERN AND EASTERN AFRICA

Jonathan Crush, Miriam Grant and Bruce Frayne

Series Editor: Prof. Jonathan Crush

African Migration and Development Series No. 3

Editorial Note

Jonathan Crush is the Director of the Southern African Migration Project (SAMP), the Director of the Southern African Research Centre (SARC) at Queen's University and an Honorary Professor at the University of Cape Town. Miriam Grant is a Professor at the University of Calgary. Bruce Frayne is a Research Fellow with the International Ford Policy Research Institute (IFPRI) and Coordinator of the Regional Network on AIDS, Livelihoods and Food Security (RENEWAL). This paper is a product of an ongoing collaboration between SAMP and IFPRI/RENEWAL funded by the IDRC. SAMP wishes to acknowledge the support of DFID. Belinda Dodson is thanked for her contribution to Section 2.1.

Published by Idasa, 6 Spin Street, Church Square, Cape Town, 8001, and Queen's University, Canada.

© Southern African Migration Project (SAMP) 2007
ISBN 1-920118-46-2

First published 2007
Produced by Idasa Publishing

Contents

Tables

Figures

1 INTRODUCTION

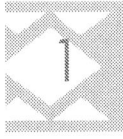

1.1 Introduction

This publication seeks to establish a background for understanding the complex and dynamic linkages between urbanization, migration, HIV/AIDS and urban food security in Southern and Eastern Africa (SEA). As urbanization accelerates, direct food transfers from rural areas are increasing as poor urban households seek to reduce their vulnerability to high food prices and a cash-intensive urban existence. At the same time, urban households or individual migrants remit money back to households in rural areas both inside and outside the country of employment. A significant proportion of remittances are used for consumption purposes, including the purchase of food.[1] These processes are underwritten by various forms of rural-urban, cross-border and circulatory migration.

Migration has clearly facilitated the rapid spread of HIV in the SEA region over the last two decades.[2] For a number of reasons, migrants and other mobile people are especially vulnerable to HIV/AIDS. The epidemic, in turn, is leading to new forms of migration, including children's migration and return migration of PLWHAs (People Living with HIV and AIDS) to rural areas.[3] Not only does this lead to a decline in remittances but it places a greater burden on rural households. Rural food production for urban household members may also be negatively affected by the impact of HIV/AIDS on rural producers. In the context of HIV/AIDS, migrants themselves may be unable to pursue other food security avenues, including urban agriculture.

As HIV/AIDS creates both short term and long term intergenerational impacts within the framework of its long wave epidemiological pattern, the development context is changing considerably. In order to formulate appro-priate policy responses, it is therefore imperative to understand the complex linkages and transfers of people and commodities which characterize the "new social economy of migration" in the SEA.[4] At the same time, it is important to understand the inter-related connections between migration and HIV/AIDS for two basic reasons. First, migrants are a particularly vulnerable group, both to HIV infection and to resultant food insecurity. Second, a disease which eats away at the fabric of the new social economy of migration will severely test the ability of urban and rural areas to provide a secure food supply for their populations, both at the aggregate and household levels.

It is against this backdrop that this publication documents the key dimen-sions of the complex connections between urbanization, migration, HIV/AIDS and food security. There is an existing and growing literature on some of these connections; between migration and HIV/AIDS, for example, and between HIV/AIDS and rural food security. However, the linkages between HIV/AIDS and urban food security are less well-established. In addition, attempts to link both HIV/AIDS and urban food security simultaneously with migration are only now being considered, and this project is the first to examine these dynamics at the regional level. That task is rendered more challenging by the fact that migration itself has been undergoing rapid changes in form over the last decade.

The publication is divided into three sections. It is designed to lay the foun-dation for further discussion and the articulation of a targeted action research agenda which addresses both the knowledge gaps and the policy and program-ming needs of the region in this field of development.

This paper begins by reviewing the literature on urbanization and migra-tion in SEA, showing how rapid urbanization is not eliminating migration but intensifying its scope and scale. The section also provides an overview of the HIV/AIDS epidemic in SEA and seeks to establish the reciprocal connections in the HIV/AIDS and migration nexus. Finally, the section reviews current evi-dence on the determinants of food security in urban areas.

The second chapter focuses on the links between migration and HIV/AIDS, migration and food security, and HIV/AIDS and food security. Research on these sets of linkage is proceeding apace although much more is known about the impact of HIV/AIDS on rural than urban food security.

The third chapter draws together these sets of relationships and outlines the key knowledge gaps and emerging research questions for the region. Although the research literature is not yet developed in this regard, various conceptual models have been devised to help understand these relationships. Although some of these models focus on rural food security and some on urban, this paper argues that the distinction is artificial, and that migration is the "missing link" between the urban and the rural. Migration links the rural and the urban social economies and emphasizes the point that urban food security cannot be isolated from rural food security and vice-versa. Finally, the paper proposes some next steps in developing a fully fledged and policy-relevant research agenda.

1.2   Urbanization and Internal Migration

Urbanization is defined as the process by which an increasing proportion of a country's population lives in urban areas over time. By this definition, Sub-Saharan Africa (SSA) is urbanizing faster than any other region. Although the urban transition has been relatively recent, more than 50% of SSA's population should be living (permanently or temporarily) in urban areas by 2030.[5] Indeed, the urban population of SSA is set to more than double between 2000 and 2020, from 217 million (34.3% of total population) to 487 million (46.2% of total population).[6] The growth in urban population in many countries of the SEA region has been dramatic between 1990 and the latest census. Although relative changes cannot be compared outright due to the variable time periods involved, rates are relatively modest for countries such as Botswana and Zambia but reach as high as 6% for Mozambique (Table 1).

As illustrated in Table 1, for selected countries of SEA, urban growth rates exceeded population growth rates for the period 1990-2003. For the 21 year period between 1982 and 2003, urbanization increased significantly in most countries, with rates more than doubling for Botswana, Kenya, Lesotho and Mozambique. This massive growth is reflected in the expansion of the number and size of mega-cities. By 2010, SSA will have at least 33 cities which exceed a million people. Metropolitan Johannesburg – the second largest mega-urban region at 3 million – will be at the core of the Gauteng region, which is expected to reach 20 million by 2020.[7]

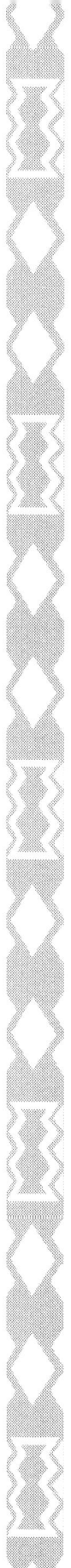

Table 1: Population and Urban Growth Rates 1990-2003 and Urbanization 1982-2003				
Country	% Population Growth Rate 1990-2003	% Urban Growth Rate 1990-2003	Urban Population (% of total) 1982	Urban Population (% of Total) 2003
Botswana	2.3	3.6	22.5	50.3
Ethiopia	2.3	4.4	10.9	16.6
Kenya	2.4	5.6	17.6	36.3
Lesotho	1.0	4.2	14.6	30.3
Madagascar	2.9	5.1	19.5	31.4
Malawi	2.0	4.4	9.6	15.9
Mozambique	2.2	6.2	14.6	35.6
South Africa	2.0	3.5	48.2	59.2
Uganda	2.9	5.3	9.2	15.3
Zambia	2.2	2.4	39.8	40.3
SSA	2.5	4.6	21.8	36
Source: Kessides[8] based on World Development Indicators 2005				

Within countries, rates of urbanization in major cities commonly exceed 4 to 5% per annum. The average primate city had annual growth rates of 5 to 6%, for example, while some saw rates of 10%, which means a doubling of city populations every ten years (less if annual increases are compounded).

There are four main drivers of urban growth in SSA: natural increase from existing urban residents; reclassification of rural as urban areas; internal rural-urban migration and international (rural-urban and urban-urban) migration. Most of the anticipated growth in the size of cities and towns over the next three decades will occur because of the transformation and reclassification of formerly "rural" settlements on the peripheries of major cities and because of natural increase within cities. Although migration is not the central driver for rapid urbanization, it plays a major role in the growth of cities as well as in strengthening the linkages between rural and urban areas and between the cities of the SEA.

Significantly, circular migration is still the dominant form of migration in most African countries. Traditional one-way movements from rural to urban destinations are much less important than circular and seasonal migration.[9] In other words, the census-based urbanization figures for countries shown in Table 1 include significant numbers of people who are living temporarily in the cities and who maintain a rural home or base which they return to on a regular basis and keep in close contact with. In West Africa, for example, Gugler recently replicated a Nigerian study he originally carried out in 1961 and found not only that urban-rural ties continue to be strong but reach beyond immediate kin to kinship groups, non-kin groups, villages and larger political entities. He argues that these ties are prevalent throughout Africa and that rural-urban migrants who maintain them and incur their costs are motivated by "present or future material rewards, political opportunities, social status and cultural commitments."[10]

In order to maintain strong social relations within the village, migrants still spend time in villages for weddings, funerals, harvests and business, followed by the necessity to spend more time in town to acquire more cash. The circular nature of this constant movement back and forth signifies "the simultaneous and overlapping presence of urban and rural spaces in migrants' lives."[11] The circular nature of rural-urban migration is also highlighted in several recent Southern African studies. In Zimbabwe, by 1994 only half as many migrants as in 1988 felt their future lay in Harare, indicating increased insecurity around urban life, employment and earning potential among in-migrants.[12] The importance of rural-urban social relations is also highlighted in Andersson's study of Buhera migrants in Harare.[13] He argues that the social security of rural-urban migrants is not spatially situated in rural agricultural production but rather socially situated in the rural-urban network. These networks are expressions of socio-cultural dispositions and are a more appropriate lens through which to view the motivation behind migration.

In Lilongwe, although rural-urban migration seldom results in permanent urban residence, migrants frequently spend periods of time in urban areas in order to improve conditions of life in villages.[14] In South Africa, one study emphasizes the resilience of urban-rural links even when the rural areas are so impoverished that they provide little by way of a livelihood for rural households.[15] In this case, migration centres on basic needs and income security, with job-related migration just one aspect of migrating families' search; infrastructure, social capital and institutional climate all influence migration demand. The results of the study indicate the instability of KwaZulu-Natal's rural population, rooted in the collapse of the natural resource base, overcrowding, violence, dispossession and hardship.

There is evidence that secondary cities have become important destinations for migrants. In Tanzania, migration during the 1980s targeted smaller towns (20,000-50,000 population) – where it was easier for urban households to secure food – over larger and primate cities.[16] Similarly, Owuor's study on urban rural-links between the secondary town of Nakuru in Kenya and its rural

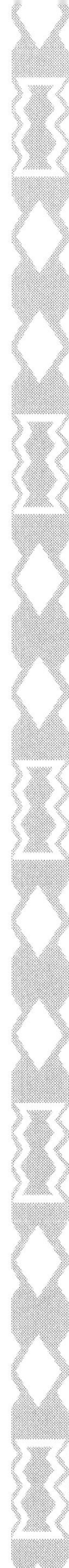

hinterland demonstrates that urban-rural linkages are not only important for rural households, but are becoming an important element of the livelihood (or survival) strategies of poorer urban households.[17]

There is also evidence that circular migration between rural and urban areas is increasing due to high costs in the city.[18] For many of the disenfranchised, such as landless peasants or those exposed to shocks of violence, depriva-tion and uncertainty, rural-rural migration is quite significant.[19] Significantly, the Namibia Migration Project found that at the national level, rural-rural migration accounted for half of all internal lifetime mobility.[20] It is important to recognize, therefore, that rural and urban boundaries are artificial distinc-tions to extended or "stretched households", who often disperse members widely to different spaces, locales and economic activities in order to support sustainable livelihoods.[21] This mobility allows individuals and families to gain new experiences and income that can be used when, where and however they decide, according to collective and individual strategies. While the household is increasingly "stretched" spatially, it is also differentiated internally, not least along gender lines.

The gendered nature of migration drivers and processes needs to be recog-nized. Internationally, the "feminization" of migration refers more to shifts in the character of women's movements, rather than a dramatic increase in num-bers (which have always been greater than traditionally recognized). In SEA, there are both qualitative and quantitative changes in internal migration under way. The absolute number of female migrants has been increasing rapidly. But the reasons for migration have also been shifting and diversifying.[22]

Gender and age are significant in migration decision-making and selectiv-ity.[23] Where home employment opportunities are limited, women may be more apt than males to migrate for employment in order to support other household members. This migration may also afford women an escape from social and family constraints and provide them with greater independence.[24] In addition, young men with limited access to family land and waged work may also be driven to migrate.[25] Within Southern Africa, for example, more women are entering the work force and more women are becoming household heads and these factors are helping to drive female migration. In South Africa, women comprised 30% of the African adult labour migration population in 1993, and this had risen to 34% by 1999. Between 1997 and the year 2000, the proportion of females among temporary migrants increased from 15% to 25% for older adult women and from 5% to 15% for young adult women – both significant increases within a short three year period.[26] The primary destina-tion for young adult women, older adult women and female children is the province of Gauteng, which is the industrial heart of South Africa. Women are also moving their families out of rural villages into nearby small towns on a permanent basis.

Data from 2002 reveals that the three main prompts for permanent internal migration of adult females are at the start or end of marriage, a move to a new dwelling for the household or a move to live with another partner.[27] The predominant driver for temporary female migration in 2002 was for work, which constituted the reason for more than 80% of moves of women aged 35 and older. Other reasons for temporary migration included for school/study and to live with another.[28] In Namibia, the increase in female migration to Windhoek over the past ten years, and the fact that urban female-headed households are poorer on average than any other household type, both indicate the feminization of rural poverty.[29]

Chronic poverty is no longer an exclusively rural problem, however, but is increasingly concentrated in urban areas. In SEA, the urban poverty rate is within 20% of the rural rate in Ethiopia, Kenya, Malawi and Mozambique. At present, at least one third or more of the urban population in Ethiopia, Kenya, Madagascar, Malawi, Mozambique and Zambia is poor.[30] Increased pauperization, combined with rapid urbanization, has created massive growth in the slum population of Sub-Saharan Africa as a whole. Between 1990 and 2001, the African urban slum population increased by 65 million, at an average annual rate of 4.5% compared with a total population growth of 2.7%. By 2001, 166.2 million people, or 72% of Sub-Saharan Africa's urban residents, were living in slums. Based on these estimates, and without effective interventions, the continent's slum population may double every 15 years, compared with a total population doubling period of 26 years.[31]

Problems of insecure tenure, overcrowding, and lack of clean water and sanitation and resultant health problems are severe and add to social and economic vulnerability of urban residents. National and municipal governments are under severe pressure to handle the implications of rapid urbanization with respect to basic service provision, housing, transportation, health care, education and employment – all of this within the constraints of economies debilitated by the impacts of structural adjustment programs, globalization, and the impact on the labour force and social systems of HIV and AIDS.

Much of the literature on internal rural-urban migration to date has concentrated on the remittance of urban goods and cash to the rural areas, with little note being taken of social linkages or rural-urban flows of cash, goods and produce.[32] From the perspective of rural livelihoods, many researchers have made the argument that environmental stress due to high population growth

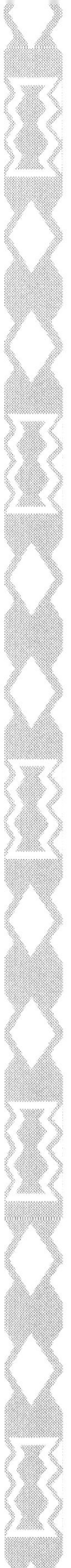

fuels rural-urban migration in the context of declining agricultural output.[33] Migration, then, is a means by which rural households can diversify their economic base.[34] The ways in which rural and urban households are mutually tied by social links and relations of reciprocity are not well-articulated in the literature.[35] The new social economy of migration needs to be better understood before the implications of HIV/AIDS for food security can be grasped.

1.3   Cross-Border Migration

SEA has a long history of cross-border intra-regional migration, dating back to the mid-nineteenth century. These movements tended to be rural-urban in character but also include urban-urban movements and, particularly in border zones, rural-rural movements. Longstanding patterns, forms, and dynamics of migration have undergone major restructuring in the last three decades with considerable implications for livelihood strategies of the poor and for poverty reduction policies. These changes include the following:

- The end of colonialism and apartheid, which were political systems designed to control internal migration and exclude most outsiders, have produced new opportunities for internal and cross-border mobility and new incentives for moving.

- SEA's integration into global and continental labour markets and trade networks has opened the region up to forms of migration commonly associated with globalization (such as temporary work schemes and skills migration.)[36]

- Growing rural poverty has pushed more people out of rural households in search of a livelihood.

- Environmental factors (including climate change, natural disasters and land degradation) continue to cause hardships and shocks which push people out of rural areas.

- Economic and political crisis and growing unemployment in some states have forced people to seek work in other countries.

- The feminization of poverty in rural SEA has produced a significant gender reconfiguration of cross-border migration streams.[37]

- The countries of the SEA have experienced recurrent waves of forced (refugee) migration over the last three decades. The cessation of threat confronts countries of origin and asylum with issues of repatriation and integration of returning migrants.

According to the latest UN estimates, there are more than 14 million international migrants in Sub-Saharan Africa. East Africa hosts 4.4 million international migrants, many of whom are refugees from Ethiopia and the Sudan.[38] Within Southern Africa, the number of foreign-born migrants in South Africa was over 1 million in 2001. Short-term legal visitors to South Africa from other Southern African Development Community (SADC) countries also increased more than tenfold after 1990 to more than seven million per year at the present time.[39]

The states of SEA are conventionally divided into migrant-origin (e.g. Mozambique, Malawi, Lesotho, Zimbabwe) and migrant-destination states (e.g. South Africa, Botswana, Namibia). In practice, most states both send and receive migrants, though in varying numbers. Several international migration streams can be identified in the SEA. All have been undergoing significant change including:

- Restructuring of traditional contract labour systems
- Growth in the volume and complexity of cross-border mobility
- Declining levels of legal migration to and within the region
- Expansion in undocumented migration and human trafficking
- Increase in skills brain drain from the region
- Large-scale resettlement and reintegration of refugees
- Feminization of cross-border migration
- Growth in intra-regional informal cross-border trade
- Rapid urbanization and growing cross-border urban-urban migrant networks

Legal and undocumented cross-border migration throughout SEA has exploded in the last decade. The pressure on limited border control resources has been enormous with long delays and inefficiency experienced at many border posts. Corruption is an endemic problem at many posts as travelers seek to bypass cumbersome and time consuming bureaucracies and gain unlawful entry. In addition, the region has experienced a major influx from other parts of the continent as well as significant growth in tourism arrivals from overseas. Intra-regional tourism has also grown to significant levels.

The reasons for the new mobility are many and varied (Table 2). The majority of intra-regional migrants to South Africa do not, contrary to popular opinion, enter to work or to look for work. Representative SAMP surveys of migrants in 6 SADC countries reveal a multiplicity of motives.[40] Cumulatively, in 6 SADC countries less than 25% went to South Africa to work or look for work. However, there was considerable inter-country variation: Mozambique (67%),

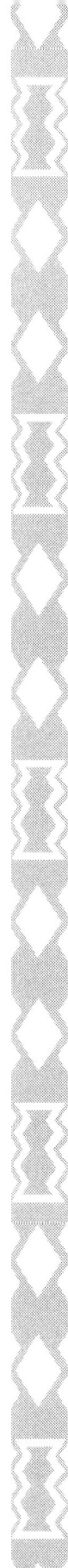

Zimbabwe (29%), Lesotho (25%), Namibia (13%) and Swaziland (9%). Other major reasons included: visiting/tourism (Namibia and Swaziland 58%), Lesotho (36%), Mozambique (17%), and Zimbabwe (16%); and trading and shopping (Zimbabwe (42%), Lesotho (22%); Swaziland (12%), Mozambique (6%), and Namibia (3%). Other reasons included to study, conduct business, and seek medical treatment.

Historically, the primary form of legal cross-border migration for employment (labour migration) in Southern Africa was male migration to the mines of South Africa, Zambia and Zimbabwe, and the commercial farms and plantations of South Africa, Swaziland and Zimbabwe. By the 1990s, only the South African gold and platinum mines continued to employ large numbers of foreign migrants; other mining sectors in South Africa (such as coal mining) and elsewhere in the region (Zambia, Zimbabwe) had moved to a local and/or more stabilized workforce.[41] During the 1990s, the South African mines experienced major downsizing and retrenchments which created considerable social disruption and increased poverty in rural supplier areas. The mines laid off local workers at a much faster rate than foreign workers. As a result, the proportion of foreign workers rose from 40% in the late 1980s to close to 60% today. This "externalization" of the workforce was particularly beneficial to Mozambique. Mozambicans now make up 25% of the mine workforce, up from 10% a decade ago (Table 3).

Table 2: Reasons for Cross-Border Migration to South Africa					
	Country of Origin				
Reason for Entry	Botswana %	Lesotho %	Mozam. %	Namibia %	Zimbabwe %
Work	7	17	45	11	15
Seek work	3	8	22	2	14
Business	6	2	2	8	7
Buy and sell goods	2	3	2	2	21
Shopping	24	19	4	1	21
Visit family	23	34	12	13	39
Medical	5	6	4	4	2
Holiday	14	2	5	19	3
Study	3	1	1	3	2
Other	12	8	2	12	3
Source: SAMP POS database at http://www.queensu.ca/samp					

Table 3: Migration to the South African Mines, 1990-2004						
Country of Origin						
Year	S.Africa	Botswana	Lesotho	Mozam.	Swaziland	Total
1990	232,338	14,497	98,788	43,951	16,618	406,192
1991	208,961	11,979	93,072	46,102	17,291	377,405
1992	185,177	12,000	92,727	49,022	16,157	355,083
1993	175,158	11,827	87,326	44,255	15,802	334,368
1994	170,876	10,939	87,248	49,250	15,101	334,414
1995	123,038	9,525	87,098	53,321	14,611	287,593
1996	126,762	9,608	80,485	54,891	14,241	285,987
1997	126,326	8,552	71,415	52,520	11,980	270,793
1998	104,483	7,229	56,132	49,507	9,518	226,869
1999	95,923	5,376	44,958	42,002	6,308	194,567
2000	95,146	5,373	50,472	44,245	8,079	203,315
2001	99,260	4,763	49,477	45,893	7,840	207,233
2002	115,824	4,227	54,154	51,355	8,697	234,257
2003	112,438	4,205	54,478	53,828	7,970	232,919
2004	120,146	3,924	48,962	48,918	7,598	180,586
Source: SAMP POS database at http://www.queensu.ca/samp						

Remittance levels have remained stable in Mozambique but fell during the 1990s to many areas, especially Lesotho, Swaziland and the Eastern Cape. This has presented a major challenge for households formerly reliant on mine remittances. Poverty levels have increased, as have domestic and family tensions. Other family members, particularly women, have begun to migrate in response. Various efforts have been made to soften the impacts of retrenchments but the overall impact has been devastating for rural areas and households once reliant on migrant remittances.

The migrant stream that attracts most public, media and official attention is "undocumented", "illegal" or "irregular" migration.[42] Irregular migration tends to be driven by economic circumstances and, in some cases, desperation. Enforcement in all countries tends to focus on identifying and deporting violators. In terms of sheer volume, South Africa is easily the regional leader, having deported over one million people since 1994.[43] Significantly, the vast majority of deportees from South Africa (upwards of 80%) are sent home to only two countries: Mozambique and Zimbabwe. Studies of sectors where irregular migrants are employed have revealed consistent violation of labour standards, sub-minimum wages, economic and sexual exploitation, and great instability and fear among migrants. These sectors include commercial agriculture in rural areas and construction, services and secondary industry in the cities.[44]

SAMP research has shown that the majority of cross-border migrants in Southern Africa are also circular migrants.[45] In other words, although many migrants stay for longer than initially intended their visits are generally temporary not permanent. Across a whole range of indices, migrants prefer living in their own countries. The major migrant-receiving countries are seen as superior only in terms of employment and economic opportunity and, sometimes, health facilities. In every other respect – personal and family safety, educational opportunities, access to land, cultural life and so on – home countries are viewed as preferable. The obvious conclusion is that economic stability and growth at home would be the single most important factor in slowing labour migration across borders.

Like internal migration, cross-border migration in Southern Africa is profoundly gendered. In the colonial period, women were generally prohibited from migrating. As the primary reason for migration in the region was wage employment, men dominated internal and cross border migration. Today women and men are differently involved in and affected by migration. Although women are increasingly part of the movement of skilled migrants within the region and out of it, and have proportionally higher educational levels than male migrants, they are more likely to be involved in less skilled and informal work. They are also more likely to be irregular migrants, with attendant disadvantages, as it is harder for them to access legal migration channels.[46] Women are migrants in their own right, as well as partners of migrant male spouses.[47]

A SAMP study found that male respondents were more likely to have been to South Africa than female (Mozambique: 41% of men and 9% of women; Zimbabwe: 25% and 20%; Lesotho: 86% and 76%).[48] But the reasons for migration tend to differ along gender lines (Table 4).

The main sectors of employment for women include agriculture (particularly seasonal work), domestic work, the service sector and trade. Men are more likely to have formal employment, particularly in the industrial (especially mining), agricultural and construction sectors. Women migrants were more likely to be disadvantaged by the migration experience than their male counterparts. They are more likely to be single or widowed, but less likely to be in formal sector employment or to own property than their male counterparts.[49] Migration is a significant livelihood strategy for women and women-headed households.[50] Although women constitute a significant part of cross border and internal migratory movement, they are also left behind as employment and earning opportunities favour men.

Table 4: Gender Differences in Migration to South Africa from 6 SADC States		
Purpose of Most Recent Visit to SA	% Males	% Females
Work	33	7
Look for work	17	3
Business	3	3
Buy and sell goods	4	10
Shop	13	23
Visit family/friends	17	38
Holiday	3	3
Medical	2	8
Other	8	5
Source: SAMP database, http://www.queensu.ca/samp		

Another particularly common, and growing, form of women's migration is motivated by opportunities for trading in other countries. Indeed, the urban areas of the SEA are being increasingly integrated into transnational continental and regional informal trade networks.[51] Informal traders or small entrepreneurs are amongst the most enterprising and energetic of contemporary migrants. Trading is a key means of livelihood for many households in some countries and needs to be better understood and, wherever possible, facilitated by policy changes governing entrance, exit and customs duties. Informal sector cross border trade is important to the transfer of goods and commodities in the region. Initial studies of informal cross-border trade in the region suggest that it:

- Is significant to the movement of food and agricultural goods in the region,

- Plays a role in regional food security,

- Plays a part in the development of small and medium enterprises,

- Is a household livelihood strategy particularly for female-headed households,

- Engages a significant number of women,

- Constitutes a significant proportion of cross-border traffic in the SADC and COMESA regions,

- Has been largely ignored by policy makers who have yet to engage with this trade.[52]

However, more needs to be known and understood about the extent of informal sector cross border trade in the region and its role in livelihood strategies and food security, and an income earning opportunity for women. Further research is required to better understand the relationship between these entrepreneurs their businesses, poverty alleviation, agricultural commodity and consumption chains and food security. Furthermore, research could inform the development of training programs to enable them to develop their businesses as well as access financial resources.

Cross-border migration has a strong relationship to poverty, social exclusion, and poverty alleviation.[53] Data on the remittance behaviour of cross-border migrants and receiving households is limited. Similarly, little information is available on their impact on national economies, economic development, inequality and financial systems in the region.[54] Furthermore, remittances in the form of goods are not recorded. Data on cash remittances is hard to gather as foreign exchange regulations, weak financial infrastructures and high transfer costs in formal systems encourage the use of informal channels for transferring money.

Despite the lack of reliable data, it is apparent that remittances to home areas do contribute significantly to household livelihoods and food security. Remittances may be in goods or cash. Remittances can play a key role in the livelihoods of migrant households allowing for social, or human capital investment in education, health and housing and food. They may also be used as capital to invest in income earning household inputs and to capitalize entrepreneurial activities.

1.4 The HIV/AIDS Epidemic

As Iliffe and Gillespie have both indicated, AIDS epidemics are multi-dimensional, long-term, phased phenomena.[55] The first wave of HIV infection is followed by a wave of opportunistic infections, tuberculosis being the most common. The onset of AIDS illness and death occurs several years later. In the final stage, depending on the prevalence of the disease and availability of treatment, there is an accumulation of macroeconomic and social impacts at household, community and national levels. At the local level, Barnett and Topouzis identify three main stages that a community may pass through: [56]

a)   AIDS initiating; with very low HIV prevalence rates and no AIDS impacts,

b)   AIDS-impending; where HIV prevalence rates are rising but most infected people are still in the asymptomatic phase before becoming ill, and

c) AIDS-impacted; when households and communities feel the impact of AIDS as infected people succumb to AIDS-related illnesses and eventually die.

In the context of the global epidemic, Africa remains the most affected region, with 25.8 million people living with HIV (Table 5). Even though Africa is home to just over 10% of the world's population, two thirds of people living with HIV are in Africa, as are 77% of all women with HIV. In 2005, an estimated 2.4 million adults and children died from AIDS-related illnesses and another 3.2 million became infected with HIV.

Table 5: HIV and AIDS in Sub-Saharan Africa, 2003-2005						
Year	Adults & children living with HIV	Adults & children newly infected with HIV	Adult preval- ence (%)	Adult & child deaths due to AIDS	No. of women (15-49) living with HIV	% HIV- infected adults (15- 49) who are female
2005	25.8 million	3.2 million	7.2	2.4 million	13.5 million	57
2003	24.9 million	3.0 million	7.3	2.1 million	13.1 million	57
Source: Compiled from UNAIDS, 2005						

Declines in adult national HIV prevalence have been recorded in just three countries: Kenya, Uganda and Zimbabwe.[57] Life expectancy for people living in eight countries (Angola, Central African Republic, Lesotho, Mozambique, Sierra Leone, Swaziland, Zambia and Zimbabwe) is forty years or less, largely due to the HIV/AIDS pandemic. In 20 countries, average citizens are poorer today than they were a decade ago and in 11 countries more people go hungry than they did a decade ago.[58]

Table 6 shows the number of persons living with HIV/AIDS and emphasizes the fact that even where prevalence rates are much lower, hundreds of thousands to millions of people are still affected. South Africa leads the way with 5.3 million persons, followed by Zimbabwe at 1.8 million, and then Tanzania, Ethiopia, Mozambique and Kenya, all of which are over 1 million, with Malawi and Zambia both approaching 1 million. Access to ARTs vary widely within each country: at least one third of those who need ART in Botswana and Uganda are receiving treatment, while in Zambia, Kenya, and Malawi 10-20% of those in need of ART were receiving it by mid-2005. Most needs went unmet. In South Africa, by mid 2005, at least 85% of those who needed ART were not receiving any, and this figure was 90% or higher for Ethiopia, Lesotho, Mozambique, Tanzania and Zimbabwe.[59]

As Table 6 shows, with the exception of Cape Town, urban HIV prevalence far exceeds national HIV prevalence and in many Eastern African countries the urban rate is two to three times the rural HIV rate. As established above, cities and towns are growing at exceptional rates, with rapid expansion of informal settlements. Hundreds of thousands of people are forced to live in conditions without basic services, security of tenure and in extreme overcrowding. These conditions enhance personal vulnerability and lead to much higher HIV prevalence.

Table 6: National and Urban HIV Prevalence in Southern and Eastern Africa, 2005			
Country	National HIV Prevalence Rate	Urban HIV Prevalence Rate	People Living With HIV/AIDS
Zimbabwe	21% (2004)	Harare 25%	1,800,000
South Africa	21.5% (2003 est.)	Cape Town 15% Durban 28%	5,300,000
Malawi	20%	Blantyre 28%	900,000
Mozambique	16%	Maputo 17.3%	1,300,000
Zambia	16.5% (2003 est.)	Lusaka 22%	920,000
Namibia	21.3% (2003 est.)	Windhoek 24%	210,000
Uganda	7%	Kampala >9%	530,000
Kenya	7%	Busia/Meru/Nakura/ Thika 9%	1,200,000
Tanzania	7%	Urban 11% (2x rural areas)	1,600,000
Rwanda	5.1% (2003 est.)	Urban 6.4% (rural 2.8%)	250,000
Burundi	6%	Bujumbura suburb 13%	250,000
Ethiopia	4.4%	Urban 12-13%	1,500,000
Somalia	0.6%	Mogadishu 0.9%	43,000
Sources: UNAIDS 2005; The World Factbook 2005.			

1.4.1   Southern Africa

Southern Africa remains the epicenter of the HIV/AIDS epidemic, with high HIV prevalence rates throughout the region, excepting Angola. The only national epidemic in the region which shows some evidence of ebbing is in Zimbabwe. Here, data from a national surveillance system shows that HIV prevalence among pregnant women dropped from 26% in 2002 to 21% in 2004 (although the role of unreliable government statistics in this decrease is not known). At 1.7 million people, and a poverty rate of 70%, the capital city of Harare has an overall HIV prevalence rate of 25%. However, HIV prevalence in women who attended antenatal or postnatal clinics dropped from 35% in 1999 to 21% in 2004 in Harare. Even though the rate of new infections could be slowing and mortality rates leveling off, 20% of pregnant women still test HIV positive and infection levels remain amongst the world's highest.[60] Nationally, life expectancy at birth dropped from 51.8 years in 1995 to 38.2 years in 2001. The WHO recently reported that Zimbabwean women now have the shortest average life expectancy in the world at 34 (compared with Zimbabwean males at 37). Although the WHO attributes this solely to HIV/AIDS, Zimbabwean doctors indicate that the failed health care system (in the midst of severe economic and political crisis) has meant that more women are dying from pregnancy and childbirth.[61]

In Bulawayo, the country's second largest city with a population close to one million, between 1990 and 2000, the overall death rate of 13.7 (per thousand population) had more than doubled, and HIV-related diseases were the leading cause of death in all age groups from 1 to 64 years.[62] Between 1995 and 2001, life expectancy in Bulawayo dropped by more than a decade from 52.4 to 41.2 years.[63]

The Zimbabwe situation has been further exacerbated by the Government's Operation Restore Order (Operation Murambatsvina), a major nationwide demolition and eviction program which started in Harare and spread to all other urban centres in 2005. With the demolition of thousands of homes, business premises and vending sites, it is estimated that 700,000 people lost their homes, their livelihoods or both, and indirectly another 2.4 million people were affected. Hundreds of thousands have been rendered homeless, without access to any basic services, and education for thousands has been disrupted. This disproportionately affected the poor and disadvantaged, who are now deeper into poverty and more vulnerable. Many of the sick, including those with HIV and AIDS, no longer have access to health care.[64] There is a major concern that increased vulnerability and population mobility, including spousal separation and livelihood insecurity, could negatively impact the HIV/ AIDS epidemic.[65]

In South Africa, HIV prevalence among pregnant women has reached its highest level yet: 29.5% of women attending antenatal clinics were HIV positive in 2004.[66] More than one in three women aged 25-34 and almost one in three women aged 20-24 were estimated to be living with HIV. The worst-affected province is KwaZulu-Natal, with a prevalence of 40%, but prevalence is also high, between 27% and 31%, in the Eastern Cape, Free State, Gauteng, Mpumalanga and North West provinces. The incredible speed of the evolution of the epidemic in South Africa – with national adult HIV prevalence at less than 1% in 1990 increasing to almost 25% by 2000, has meant a concomitant increase in mortality: Death rates of those 15 years and older increased by 62% from 1997-2002 and deaths in the 25-44 age group more than doubled during that time. At present, South Africa experiences an estimated 900 deaths a day from the epidemic.[67] Urban HIV prevalence rates cover a wide range: Cape Town (population 2 million) has a prevalence of 15% while Durban (population of 3 million) has a 28% prevalence rate. The Actuarial Society of South Africa estimates that it will be another 10 years before the pandemic breaks.[68]

Exceedingly high prevalence rates – often over 30% for pregnant women – are still recorded in Botswana, Lesotho, Namibia and Swaziland. In Swaziland, HIV prevalence among pregnant women increased from 34% in the year 2000 to 43% in 2004. Prevalence is even higher at 56% among pregnant women in the 25-29 year old group. Within Swaziland, there is little regional variance in HIV prevalence among pregnant women and the overall national HIV prevalence is 39%.[69] In Lesotho, HIV prevalence is 27% amongst antenatal clinic attendees, down slightly from 29% in 2003.[70] National HIV prevalence has reached 31%. Botswana also has a national prevalence rate of 39%, although national prevalence among pregnant women has remained between 35% and 37% since 2001, which may indicate some stabilization. For pregnant women 25 years and older, prevalence soared to 43% in 2003.[71]

Malawi experiences wide regional variation in prevalence from 7% in the central region to 33% at the southern tip, with national prevalence around 20%. Two negative trends here are increasing prevalence at rural clinics and rising prevalence amongst young pregnant women (15% for 15-19 year olds and 20% for 20-24 year olds).[72] In Blantyre, with a population which exceeds 700,000 and an urban poverty rate of 54%, the HIV prevalence rate is 28%.[73]

The epidemic in Mozambique is increasing, with rising levels in all regions and an estimated increase in national adult HIV prevalence from 14% to slightly above 16% in the 2002-2004 period. In the capital city, Maputo, with a population of 966,837, HIV prevalence is 17.3%. Population migration and mobility is a driving force, since HIV is spreading faster in provinces which have main transport links with Malawi, South Africa and Zimbabwe. High infection rates are also evident in Gaza province, which borders Zimbabwe and South Africa, and is a major source of migrants for South African industry and farms, and in Sofala province, which is divided by Zimbabwe's main export route.[74]

In Zambia, HIV prevalence among 15-44 year old pregnant women has remained at 18-20% since 1994. However, rising prevalence for 15-19 year-olds attending antenatal clinics between 1998 and 2002 indicate that new infections continue to occur at significant rates. In the capital city of Lusaka (population 1.6 million), there is a 52% urban poverty rate and an HIV prevalence of 22%. Altogether, urban residents are twice as likely as rural residents to be infected with HIV. The highest levels of infection are once again tied to population mobility and are tied to cities and towns situated along major transport routes. This includes Kabwe, Kapiri, Mposhi, Livingstone and Ndola, where 22-32% of pregnant women were HIV positive in 2002.[75]

Angola has the lowest HIV prevalence rate within the region with an esti-mated 2.8% of pregnant women testing positive. However, the capital city of Luanda had reached a prevalence of 4.4% in 2004. A prevalence rate of 33% has been found amongst commercial sex workers, indicating potential for major epidemic growth.[76] The highest prevalence is located in the two provinces of Cunene and Kuando-Kubango, both of which share a border with Namibia, in a region where migration is significant.[77]

There is considerable geographical variation in levels of HIV prevalence in Namibia, from 8.5% in Opuwo in the remote northwest, to 42% in Katima Mulilo, which is situated in the Caprivi strip which borders Angola, Botswana and Zambia, an area of high mobility. Some parts of Namibia therefore experi-ence rates equivalent to the worst hit areas of Swaziland, Botswana and South Africa. The mobility of the mining and fishing labour force results in high rates in the coastal towns of Luderitz, Swakopmund and Walvis Bay (22%-28%).[78] Windhoek, the capital city (population 233,000) has a prevalence rate of 24%, and has experienced dramatic in-migration since independence in 1990, as illustrated in the graph below (Figure 1).

Figure 1: Rural-Urban Migration Trend for Windhoek: 1944-2000

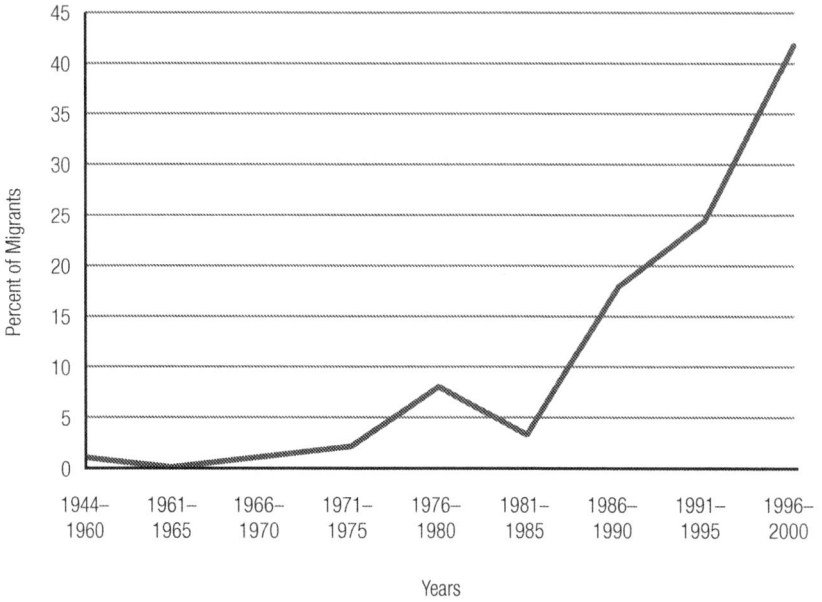

Source: Frayne, B. 2001, note 4.

HIV/AIDS in Urban Southern Africa

Southern Africa has the highest HIV prevalence rates in the world. It is also home to 30% of all global persons living with HIV/AIDS. Botswana and Swaziland have the highest prevalence rates in the world at 39% and the only country that has shown any decrease in prevalence has been Zimbabwe, although these figures are questionable and also predate the impact of Operation Restore Order. HIV prevalence in urban areas is higher than national prevalence levels as are regions along borders and transport routes which experience high levels of mobility. These serious national AIDS epidemics are set to continue for some time.

1.4.2   East Africa

Turning to East Africa, although national prevalence within Uganda peaked at over 15% in the early 1990s, this has declined and may be the result of a major national campaign. At present, national prevalence lies at 7%, although it rises to 10% for Ugandans in the 30-39 year group. In urban areas in

Uganda, HIV prevalence among women was almost twice as high as men (13% versus 7.3%). Overall infection rates were highest for the capital city of Kampala (population 1.2 million) at more than 9%, and for the Central and North-Central regions.[79] Little is documented about the effect of conflict on HIV prevalence rates; however, there is currently a RENEWAL study underway in Uganda which examines the situation of internally displaced people in the refugee camps.[80] Moreover, the continued conflict in northern Uganda may contribute to a renewed increase of HIV and AIDS in the country, particularly amongst children and women.

Kenya's epidemic peaked in the late 1990s with a national adult prevalence of 10%, which dropped to 7% in 2003. Infection levels for urban residents peaked in the mid 1990s, prior to that of rural residents, which later dropped but at a slower rate than urban areas. Kenya has the distinction of being only the second SSA country whose national HIV infection rates have declined steadily. The clearest example of this turnaround has been amongst pregnant women in the urban centres of Kenya – especially in Busia, Meru, Nakaru and Thika – where HIV prevalence dropped from 28% in 1999 to 9% in 2003. There have also been falls in other urban areas, including the capital, Nairobi (population between 3 and 4 million). The decline in Kenya's national prevalence rates can be attributed to several factors, including behavioural change, the mature stage of the epidemic where death rates can exceed new infection rates, and the deaths of the more at-risk population which removes them from the transmission circuit.[81] While these declines appear remarkable in the broader regional context, it is important to emphasize that in Kenya, as elsewhere, prevalence rates vary significantly across the country, potentially masking hard-hit communities who may be bypassed by interventions as a result.[82] For example, the fishing communities of the Lake Victoria Basin have a lifestyle that exposes them to viral transmission and their prevalence rates of 31% are testimony to this. Similarly disproportionate prevalence rates have been recorded among fisherfolk in the adjacent countries of Tanzania and Uganda.[83]

Although the prevalence rate in mainland Tanzania is fairly low at 7%, it is twice as high in urban (11%) than in rural areas. Altogether, it is estimated that 1.5 million people are living with HIV/AIDS. Although 12 years ago ante-natal clinic HIV prevalence reached 20% in Mbeya and 36% at some clinics, it now appears to have stabilized. Antenatal infection rates have declined in Dar es Salaam and Mtware since 2002, but they have risen in the capital city of Dodoma (population over 300,000). However, according to a recent survey in rural parts of the country, 40% of married men admitted to having

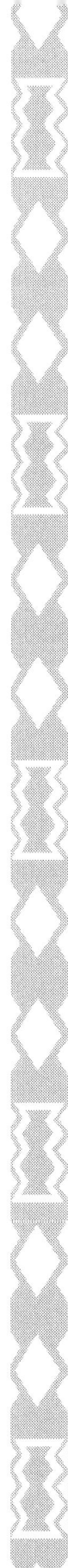

extramarital affairs which presents an alarming trend for the possibility of new infections.[84]

Urban areas in Rwanda also mirror patterns found elsewhere, with prevalence twice as high as for rural areas (6.4% median prevalence in 2003 compared with 2.8% for rural areas) and with the capital city of Kigali (2005 population of 851,024) the worst hit. HIV prevalence fluctuations range widely in Burundi, from 2% in Kiremba to 13% in a suburb of the capital city of Bujumbura with an estimated national prevalence rate of 6%.[85]

Urban HIV prevalence rates in Addis, Ethiopia, are almost three times the national level of an estimated 4.4%. Pregnant women in towns and cities have had HIV prevalence rates between 12 and 13% since the mid 1990s. However, with 85% of the population situated in rural areas, more people in rural areas are now being infected than in urban, with rural prevalence increasing from 1.9% in 2000 to 2.6% in 2003.[86] While this may be the trend, rural poverty is chronic, severe and in many cases worsening with time, raising general vulnerability to HIV and AIDS through poverty mitigation (usually survival) behaviours involving mobility. For example, women and girls, facing destitution from asset losses, move to towns to begin making a living in the commercial sex worker industry and expose themselves to HIV.[87] The challenges facing Ethiopia are significant: there are more than 1.5 million people living with HIV (2004) and more than 4.5 million orphans, of whom at least 500,000 are AIDS orphans. AIDS caused an estimated 30% of deaths in 2003, and in mid-2005, fewer than 10% of people who needed ART were receiving it.[88] Deaths due to AIDS have already brought down life expectancy which was expected to fall by 4.6 years in 2003.[89] It is noteworthy that in terms of disease stage and prevalence rates, Ethiopia is now where South Africa was in 1994.

HIV prevalence rates are low for both Eritrea and Somalia. In 2003, Eritrea had a low national adult prevalence of 2.4%, with regional ranges from under 2% to more than 7%. In Somalia, a 2004 national survey of pregnant women recorded an average rate of 0.6%, with the highest infection rates found in the capital city of Mogadishu (0.9%).[90] With 7% of women attending one clinic in Mogadishu found to be HIV positive, it appears that urban concentration is once again the dominant pattern. Knowledge of HIV transmission is very low, which indicates the need for a prevention and education program, but in societies where sexuality and sexual practices are not openly discussed, such programs face significant obstacles.

Urban HIV in Eastern Africa

National adult HIV prevalence rates are much lower in East African countries compared with Southern African countries although HIV prevalence
rates still remain high. Cities and towns tend to exceed national and rural
prevalence rates. Although epidemics appear to be stable, they remain
serious and will continue for many years to come. Socio-economic and
socio-cultural factors which create and enhance vulnerability need to be
addressed.

1.5   Determinants of Urban Food Security

The right to food has been recognized by various international declarations,
including the Universal Declaration of Human Rights.[91] Food security is usually defined as "access by all people at all times to sufficient food for an active
healthy life."[92] Definitions of food security usually include food supply, access,
adequacy, utilization, safety and cultural acceptability of food for all people at
all times.[93] Barrett outlines four major elements of a useful operational concep-
tion of food security:[94]

*   the physiological needs of individuals (nutritional requirements and
    energy expenditure levels);

*   the complementarities and tradeoffs among food and other basic neces-
    sities (most notably health care and education, among other things);

*   changes over time, and people's perceptions of and responses to these
    changes (for example, consumption smoothing) and, especially;

*   uncertainty and risk (vulnerability, and people's perceptions and respons-
    es to risk).

Food security is no longer viewed as a failure to produce enough food nationally, but rather as a failure of livelihoods to provide an adequate supply at
the household level.[95] Dowler maintains that food insecurity is a synonym for
food poverty, which reflects the fact that food insecurity goes beyond physical
efficiency of food consumption to include the ability "to acquire or consume
an adequate quantity or quality of food in socially acceptable ways, or the
uncertainty that one will be able to do so."[96] These conceptions are reflected
in factors which help to measure the degree of food insecurity. A population or
livelihood group is considered acutely food insecure if:

*   people experience a large reduction in their major source of food and are

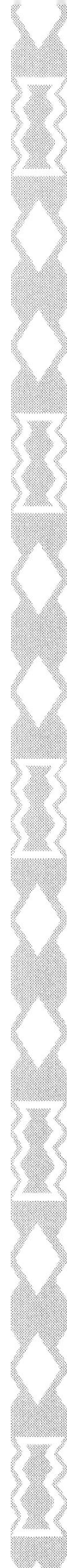

unable to make up the difference through new strategies;

- the prevalence of malnutrition is abnormally high for the time of year, and this cannot be accounted for by either health or care factors;

- a large proportion of the population or group is using marginal or unsustainable coping strategies; and

- people are using 'coping' strategies that are damaging their livelihoods in the longer term, or incur some other unacceptable cost, such as acting illegally or immorally.[97]

Sub-Saharan Africa is the only region in the world where the number of people who live in extreme poverty has almost doubled over the last two decades: from 164 million in 1981 to 314 million today.[98] Chronic urban poverty is critically linked with urban food insecurity. As urban areas within SEA grow at unprecedented rates, the infrastructure and tax bases of cities cannot meet the increased demands for services and this has led to increased crowding and a deteriorating urban environment.[99] This means that access to health care, water, housing and education are all problematic.[100]

Levels of urban poverty appear to be increasing in much of Africa. Unemployment and underemployment are characteristic of urban economies which have been in decline since the 1970s and 1980s, exacerbated by rapid urbanization rates.[101] Cities and towns are cash-intensive and residents often have to pay for goods and services (such as fuel and housing) that they do not have to pay for in rural areas. High costs for non-food essentials means that urban dwellers spend a smaller proportion of their incomes on food because they must pay for goods such as housing, energy, transportation, household items, education, health care and personal items.[102] Also, prices vary not just between rural and urban areas but also between urban areas.

As poor households struggle to meet urban expenses, the type, quantity and quality of food consumption tends to be an area of cut-back since it is not viewed as a fixed, absolute expense. Thus, households are thrust into food insecurity. Kironde, for example, found that in Tanzania the income needed for 2000 calories per day was 19.7% higher in towns (excluding Dar es Salaam) than rural areas and 98.2% higher in Dar than in rural areas.[103] Many recent urban poverty assessment studies reaffirm this trend. For example, in Accra, Maxwell et al found that urban households buy more than 90% of their food and 40% of households could be classified as insecure with respect to calorie intake. In low-income settlements in Dhaka, for sake of comparison, 50% of the population was below the chronic poverty line and 42% was below a local line of minimum food plus 20% for basic necessities.[104]

The analysis of food insecurity is usually focused upon risk factors and whether households can cope with shortfalls. In the city, this revolves around access to cash for food and basic necessities, which is tied directly to wages and prices, but also includes factors such as overcrowding, an unhygienic environment and the lack of a functional safety net.[105]

Food prices are integral to the food security of urban dwellers. Urban retail markets in most developing cities are small and scattered, and although this may not be efficient, they do serve the needs of the poor, who are forced to buy food every day and in small quantities since they lack the cash to buy in bulk. For many years, food prices in urban areas were kept cheap through subsidies, overvalued exchange rates and trade restrictions. However, structural adjustment programmes during the 1980s and 1990s reversed these policies and led to food prices that often increased much faster than wages.[106] The urban poor are further hampered by their dependence on low wage, casual, temporary or seasonal work and thus their cash flows are intermittent and influx, which directly impacts upon their ability to buy food.

In Southern Africa, in particular, many people are undernourished due to poor quality diets and infections. A poor diet usually means inadequate quantities of protein, carbohydrates and micronutrients which are all necessary for various human functions. Pregnant women who live in environments which lack iodine need to consume iodized salt for the normal development of the foetal brain. In addition, if people do not consume enough fruits and vegetables, deficiencies in vitamins A, C and other nutrients make them more susceptible to disease.[107] Research in many developing countries shows that poor nutrition leads to reduced productivity.[108] A recent study by the International Food Policy Research Institute (IFPRI) in 15 developing countries revealed that poverty and malnutrition increase along with urbanization. Using WHO data, the study found that the urban share of underweight children increased in 11 of the 15 countries and the absolute number increased in 9 of the 15 countries.[109]

Children are particularly vulnerable to the effects of malnutrition and malnourishment. Malnutrition in the form of stunted and underweight children worsened in South Africa during the late 1990s.[110] A recent UNICEF study of childhood nutritional status in Southern Africa over a ten year period showed deterioration in conditions in Zimbabwe and Zambia in 2001-2003. Overall, 2.3 million children were underweight in the 6 countries studied, with more than 30% of children in Malawi and Mozambique showing stunted growth. In all countries except Lesotho and Swaziland, urban and peri-urban areas started with the lowest levels of underweight children but deteriorated the most over the ten years, while most rural areas tended to improve.[111]

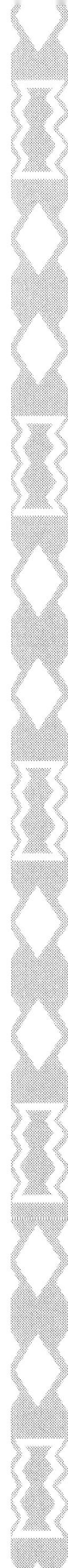

Although African cities are growing at an unprecedented rate and urban poverty is back on the agenda with respect to both research and donor priorities, Maxwell contends that urban food security has become politically invisible. He cites several reasons for this:[112]

- urban food security is fairly invisible to urban planners and managers as they scramble to deal with more urgent visible political issues such as unemployment, the informal sector, overcrowding, decaying infrastructure and declining services – even though food security and malnutrition are all linked to these other problems;

- unless there are major problems with food supply or sudden increases in food prices, food insecurity rarely becomes a political issue and therefore is dealt with at the household level; and

- development theory has reinforced the notion that food insecurity and poverty are generally rural problems.

One aspect of urban food security which has largely been ignored in the literature is that of urban food remittances from extended and immediate family in the rural areas. Frayne explores this issue in Namibia, and finds that rural sources of food are important for migrant and non-migrant households alike in the context of limited employment and high rural-urban migration.[113] In this study, 66% of Windhoek households had received food over the past year from friends and relatives in the rural areas and 58% were sent food from 2-6 times in the past year.

The reciprocity between rural and urban households is key here, with urban households sending cash remittances to rural families in the semi-subsistence sector which drives the purchase of food and other necessities in the rural areas and thereby contributes to the availability of a 'rural surplus' for remitting to the urban household. Thus, social networks are the infrastructure that enables the flow of goods between rural and urban areas.[114] However, there are gender differences in amounts and types of food received and for women it is the lack of well-established links to the north as well as rights to land that account for the fact that they receive smaller amounts of food.

Potts also found in Zimbabwe that households which have access to rural production are remitting increasing amounts of food to urban areas.[115] In addition, Oucho reports that it is usually rural households with access to urban remittances who are the most productive farmers in East Africa, which may apply to Southern Africa. In his study, Oucho found that 48% of urban remittances are used either to buy or improve land and that the strength of ties between rural and urban households stimulates the rural economy at both household and community levels.[116]

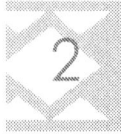

2 MAKING THE LINKAGES

2.1 Migration and HIV/AIDS[117]

Links between HIV/AIDS and migration are complex.[118] The highest incidence of HIV/AIDS is in the SEA countries with good transport infrastructure, relatively high levels of economic development, and highly mobile populations. Migration is tied to the rapid spread and high prevalence of HIV/AIDS in the following ways:

* Migrant communities are socially and economically marginalized and have high rates of infection;

* Migrant social and sexual networks make them more vulnerable to infection;

* Migration encourages high-risk sexual behaviour;

* Migrants are harder to reach for preventive education, condom provision, HIV testing and treatment and care.[119]

The incidence of HIV is generally higher among migrants and the sexual partners of migrants.[120] The infection rate is very high amongst truck drivers – over 90% reported in one South African study.[121] Border towns have high HIV prevalence, as places where truck drivers encounter stable local populations, and are removed from AIDS intervention programs.[122] Refugees and internally-displaced persons are also especially vulnerable to HIV infection.

In linking human mobility and the epidemiology of HIV/AIDS, it is important to note that different forms of migration lead to different social and geographical forms of migrant 'community', and thus to different causes and cultures of risk. Where single-sex labour migration is regularized and formalized as in the South African mines, migrant communities and an associated migrant culture has developed.[123] Sex and sexuality are integral components of such cultures, including commercial or 'transactional' sex and heterosexual as well as homosexual relations, in addition to sex with a female partner at 'home.' Other forms of mobility disrupt or prevent the formation of any stable, place-based community. People who have multiple 'homes', or who spend a lot of their time away from or between homes, lead lives of contingent encounters and short-term relationships, whether economic, social or sexual. This encourages high-risk sexual behaviour, including obtaining sex on a commercial basis. For example, in Zambia, low-income men living away from home for one or more months per year are more than twice as likely to die as men living at home.[124] While 'on the road,' women especially are vulnerable to exploitation and harassment, which can include sexual assault. In Malawi, poor women and girls who undertake cash-earning piecemeal work (ganyu) beyond the confines of the village are particularly at risk as transactional sex is increasingly incorporated into ganyu contracts.[125] The gender dynamics of migration therefore lead to differences between men and women in terms of their risk of exposure to HIV.[126]

HIV/AIDS is also becoming an increasingly important cause of migration and mobility. For example:

- People with AIDS commonly return to live with family members to obtain care;

- Loss of income though death or debilitation of a migrant encourages migration by other household members;

- HIV/AIDS can lead to a decline in rural productivity and food security, increasing pressure for out-migration;

- Replacement of migrant workers with HIV/AIDS with new migrant workers;

- Migration to avoid stigmatization;

- Migration to obtain health care;

- Skills gaps and shortages could prompt countries to seek replacement skills from other countries;

- AIDS orphans (who may themselves be HIV positive) migrate to live with relatives or to seek their own income-earning opportunities;[127]

- New widows or widowers (also themselves often HIV positive) may migrate upon the death of their partner.

In drawing attention to the connections between HIV/AIDS and human mobility, it is essential not to "stigmatize" migrants as bearers of disease, as people to be 'kept out' by implementing stricter migration controls. Xenophobia further marginalizes already-vulnerable migrant communities and exacerbates the socio-economic conditions that contribute to the spread of HIV. Likewise, legal restrictions that attempt to prevent migration create clandestine flows of people, excluded from access to social and medical services. Instead of futile attempts to prevent people from moving, there need to be HIV/AIDS interventions, from education and prevention through testing and counseling to treatment and care, that are designed for and targeted at particular migrant populations.

There are at least four broad categories of mobile population, each demanding a different form of response:

- Migrant or immigrant communities of people who have left one place to settle in another, either long-term or permanently. They require focused interventions in their new location until such time as they become fully integrated into their new societies;

- Trans-migrants who have 'homes' in more than one location. They require interventions at both 'homes' as well as in transit;

- Itinerant or mobile populations, who either have no 'home' or who spend most of their time away from home (truckers, seafarers, CSWs, construction workers). Perhaps the most difficult to reach, as they do not constitute a spatially fixed community, these people require interventions that mirror their movements, for example condoms at truck stops, education material on buses, mobile clinics and so on;

- Temporarily displaced communities such as refugees and internally displaced persons. Interventions require rapid response in highly mobile form, especially in conditions where the very circumstances forcing people to move, such as war, simultaneously expose them to the threat of HIV infection.

Infusing migrant communities with education, prevention, testing, treatment and care is the only realistic means of dealing with the current HIV/AIDS epidemic and containing its further spread. To further stigmatize or marginalize migrants, or even to ignore their particular HIV/AIDS intervention needs, serves only to strengthen the dangerous synergy between HIV/AIDS and migration.

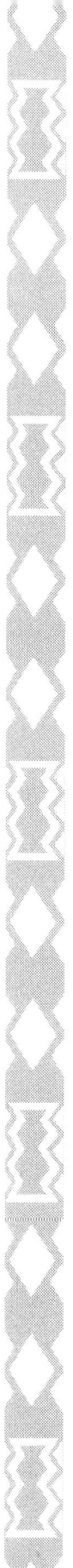

2.2   Migration and Food Security

Impacts of out-migration on source areas vary considerably. Migration can be a response to poverty but, as Skeldon notes, the extremely poor are generally excluded from migration opportunities. While migration may reduce poverty it almost always enhances inequality, since migration is a selective process.[128] The major issue is what opportunities are available to which groups and whether the type of migratory work benefits migrants and their families by improving their assets and human capital.[129]

The links between migration and food security specifically need to be viewed at two levels. First, at a more general level, there is the question of whether migration facilitates or undermines the overall food security of rural and urban populations. Second, there is the more specific question of the food security of migrants themselves and how this is secured.

As indicated above, flows of migrants are increasingly complex. In general, however, households in SEA use migration as a survival and accumulation strategy, along with income diversification. Krokfors views migration as a response to poverty and environmental stress, and uses the term 'multi-active households' to describe households which engage in different income generating activities.[130] One characteristic of these changes is risk spreading or risk management on the part of households as they engage in multiple modes of livelihood to improve their standard of living or to just survive. Jamal and Weeks refer to this as the 'trader-cum-wage earner-cum-shamba growing' class.[131] Tacoli notes emerging higher levels of multi-activity, notably among younger generations, and an increase in mobility accompanied by strong social and economic links with home areas. Typically, therefore, households are now spatially "stretched" between rural and urban areas.

There is now what Frayne terms a 'complex system of cyclical or reciprocal migration between rural and urban areas.' This has led to an increased inter-dependency of rural and urban systems and 'reciprocal urbanization' where movement of people and goods back and forth is supported by enhanced communications and transportation.[132] Owuro postulates that the terms 'multi-spatial households' and 'multiple-home households' are not as appropriate as 'multi-spatial livelihoods' since different income-generating activities in different geographical locales does not necessarily imply a divided household. 'Multi-spatial livelihood' means that a household has both urban and rural sources of food and income.[133] In one study of households with multi-spatial livelihoods, households which combined crop production with marketing, and several non-farm and off-farm income-generating activities were found to be the most successful economically and the most food secure.[134]

The impact of migration on rural agriculture is also a key consideration.[135] The relationship is complicated by numerous other factors. De Haan, for example, notes that the impact is dependent on "the context, on seasonality of movement, educational levels of migrants, the length of time spent away, assets, and social structures and institutions allowing – in case of single male migration – women and others to pursue activities previously reserved for men and household heads."[136] Logically, if migration deprives rural areas of labour and impacts negatively on production, then it is likely to increase the food insecurity of rural populations. In Central Mali, for example, absent young men were sorely missed, especially by the smallest households, and remittances were seen as poor substitutes for young men's labour.[137] In a Malawi study, 45% of women were performing tasks once handled by men, but women were quite over-burdened and did not receive enough remittances to hire labour.[138] In his study on migration and food security in Namibia, Frayne identifies distress migration where children from urban homes are sent to stay with relatives elsewhere because households did not have enough money to support the children in Windhoek. Another form of distress migration is to send adult members to the rural areas, either as returnees or new migrants in situations where few in the household are employed. This reduces the need for the urban household to "ration food, sell assets, borrow food or money, or engage in crime to survive."[139]

The picture is further complicated by two factors: first, absent migrants are not food consumers which may decrease the pressure on the consumption levels of the household. Second, migrants who have gainful employment or other income-generating activity in town commonly send remittances home. There is some evidence that remittances from urban to rural areas are declining.[140] But the fundamental question is what rural households do with remittances in cash and kind. Are these remittances invested in rural agriculture and other productive income-generating activity? The evidence from a recent study by SAMP of remittance usage in 6 SADC countries found that in general they are not. Looking at household averages for all countries, food and groceries are by far the most important (93% of households) followed by transportation (44%), fuel (44%), utilities (38%), education (31%) and medical expenses (30%). Certain categories of expenses are more important in certain countries. Education (primarily school fees) is important in Zimbabwe (57% of households) and Mozambique (44%); medical expenses are important in Zimbabwe (40%), Swaziland (39%) and Mozambique (31%); and savings are important in Zimbabwe (36%) and Botswana (28%). Housing is a major category only in Zimbabwe (46%); as is clothing in Lesotho (73%) and Zimbabwe (54%); and

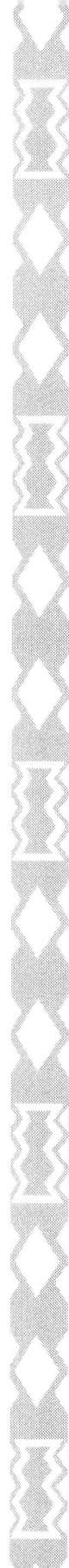

farming expenses in Swaziland (39%). This tends to confirm other evidence that women in Swaziland were able to increase agricultural production through a combination of remittances from absent males and through government provision of a tractor-rental service.[141]

When the amount spent by category is compared across countries, the largest amounts were spent on building (R576), farming (R434), clothes (R267), food (R288), and special events (R239). Building is the largest median expense category in all five countries with food expenses second in Lesotho (R400) and Mozambique (R251), third in Botswana (R346), fourth in Zimbabwe (R64) and fifth in Swaziland (R300). However, looking only at the amount spent on such items as building and special events skews the picture because these expenses affect relatively few households. When the weighted value of expenditure items is compared, the major importance of food as an expense category is revealed. It is the most important expense item in all five countries. The three most important items by country in 1000s of rands are: Botswana: food (R186), clothes (R33), fuel (R31); Lesotho: food (R377), clothes (R371), special events (R75); Mozambique: food (R124), clothes (R24), building (R22); Swaziland: food (R281), farming (R232), education (R116); and Zimbabwe: food (R40), education (R18), building (R15). Depending on the country, between 2 and 6 times more money is spent on food than the next most important expense item which highlights the importance of the food expense for migrant-sending households. In other words, the evidence to hand suggests that migrant remittances are not generally invested in farming but used primarily to purchase food to increase the food security of rural household members.

As noted above, there is scattered evidence from throughout SEA that food transfers from rural to urban areas are well-established and even increasing in volume. Frayne, for example, found that the percentage of urban households which received food regularly was higher than the percentage of those who remitted cash to rural extended family members. In Harare, Drakakis-Smith reported that 20% of respondents received gifts of food from rural areas.[142] In Dakar, Senegal, there was also a considerable flow of both food and cash from rural to urban homes.[143] In Kenya, rural crop cultivation far exceeded urban cultivation in its contribution to the energy requirements of urban residents in Nakuru.[144] This research supports the general tenet that transfers of food, and sometimes cash, from rural to urban areas are on the increase and that the balance of favour is moving to the urban side.

The second area of focus in unraveling the connections between migration and food security concerns the situation of migrants themselves. Does migration itself have a positive or negative impact on the access of migrants in urban areas to quality food? This question requires much further research. One area which has received some attention is the issue of urban food production (or urban agriculture). Within urban and peri-urban areas, there has been an increase in urban agriculture (UA) since the late 1970s. As real wages have declined over time, and as imported food prices have risen, many urban residents have turned to UA. Ellis and Sumberg[145] summarize the reasons for engaging in UA as follows:

- as a means of survival for the very poor;

- as a personal strategy for women to meet part of family food security needs in the context of insufficient, uncertain or unstable cash allocations by male wage earners within the household;[146]

- as a contribution to food security in general;

- as a substitute for cash purchases of food, especially for higher priced food such as eggs, meat, milk, fruit and vegetables so that cash can be used for other items;[147]

- as a means to supplement cash earnings of the family and meet other objectives such as children's schooling;[148]

- as a commercial rather than subsistence activity.

Many engage in UA for a combination of reasons and these are not mutually exclusive. Some studies have found that many high and middle-income households tend to engage in UA, usually for commercial reasons. In a study based on Gabarone, Hovorka makes the argument that UA plays a very important entrepreneurial role which increases the agency of urban dwellers.[149] In Nairobi, Freeman finds that UA is dominated by women who are divided into those who farm for subsistence and those who farm for cash income.[150] However, poorer households, which include newly arrived migrants, are often excluded from access to land due to both formal and informal gatekeeping within the city.[151] The question therefore arises as to the extent to which migrants participate in UA and its benefits.

In general, rural-urban migration has been thought to improve the personal food security of the individual migrant. In some sectors, such as mining and plantation agriculture, this is clearly the case. The mines and estates have an interest in maintaining a well-fed workforce and provide regular and nutritious meals as a supplement to wages. Similarly, migrants in the services sector are likely to have access to cheap, good quality food. On the other hand, migrants working in sectors such as construction and industry may have to spend a disproportionate part of their wage envelope on food. Migrants in employment or self-employment are certainly not individual consumers. Many have depend-

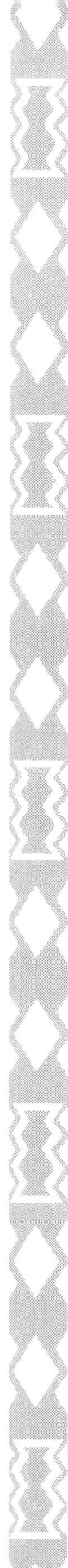

ents in urban areas and pool resources into a "common pot" to sustain the urban half of the split household (or a separate urban household with another partner and dependents). Although migrants are largely dependent on cash purchases for food, urban food prices (particularly where there is a thriving informal sector) may be lower than in rural areas. However, the evidence suggests that poor urban households, including migrants, spend a disproportionate amount of their income on food. If there is strong pressure to remit, they may be more vulnerable to going short themselves.

New forms of urbanization and migration are clearly emerging. They reflect complex demographic, social and commodity exchanges, based on reciprocity and reciprocal migration. Food transfers are vital to urban food security at the household level. Remittance transfers are equally vital to food security in many rural areas. Households with weak ties to rural families and without access to rural land to cultivate, including the poorest urban households and some female headed households, are the most vulnerable to deprivation and generally live under severe risk of hunger.

2.3   HIV/AIDS and Food Security

At a biological level, macro- and micro-nutrients play a critical role in the immune response to infectious diseases and survival. Since HIV directly attacks the immune system, HIV and malnutrition work in tandem:

> HIV compromises nutritional status and this in turn increases susceptibility to opportunistic infections. Malnutrition, on the other hand, exacerbates the effects of HIV by further weakening the immune system. Clinical studies show that HIV disease progression is more rapid in individuals with compromised nutrition.[152]

Within HIV-affected households, there is increased risk of food insecurity and malnutrition as sick members are unable to work, income declines, expenditure on health care increases, care-giving burdens increase and there is less time for looking after children.[153] The concept of nutrition security has also come forward as a key dimension in the prevention, care, treatment and mitigation of HIV/AIDS. A household can be viewed as nutrition secure when access to a variety of food is accompanied by a sanitary environment, adequate health services and adequate care to ensure a healthy life for all household members.[154]

At the community level, because HIV/AIDS strikes the most economically active and because it is so widespread, the impact is not just across sectors, but significantly systematic.[155] In assessing the impact on agriculture, the FAO suggests that if four people for each of the 42 million people living with HIV are impacted, the virus will affect 160 million globally. The resulting humanitarian crisis would be especially acute in Southern Africa, where many countries have prevalence rates over 17%. By 2020, Namibia could lose up to 26% of its agricultural force due to HIV/AIDS, Zimbabwe 23%, Mozambique and South Africa 20% and Malawi 14%.[156] Table 7 shows the impacts HIV/AIDS has on agricultural systems and household food security.

Table 7: Common Impacts of HIV/AIDS on Agriculture	
How HIV/AIDS changes the context of agricultural growth	Leads to:
Labour changes:	Less land being farmed
Shortage of household labour due to:	Underfarming of land
Mortality	More child labour
Surviving adults doing care-giving	Less labour-intensive crops grown
Shortage of hired labour due to:	Emphasis on small livestock and cash crops
Mortality	Greater emphasis on small livestock cultivation
Migration to cities	Decline in marketed output for crop processors
Lack of cash to pay for it	Natural resource mining (the future is heavily discounted)
Loss of farm-specific knowledge:	
Premature mortality curtails period for intergenerational role modeling and knowledge transfer	Less appropriate farming practices within a more hostile farming environment
	More inexperienced farmers who need training, role models (e.g. youth)
Income changes:	
Fewer earners, increase in dependency ratio	More off-farm income sources
Greater expenditure on medical, transport, special needs of ill	Migration
Institutional and organizational changes:	
Loss of institutional knowledge, high turnover, low investment in staff development	Weaker rural institutions (e.g. extension services, microfinance institutions, NGOs)
	Weaker social capital
	Weakening of property rights for some
	Weakening of asset base of women (especially land)
Source: Haddad and Gillespie (2005)[157]	

As Table 7 illustrates, the impact of HIV/AIDS is not only immediate, but cumulative and far-reaching. As social capital erodes, youth are left untrained and unprepared for agricultural production and decisions related to the future. The average life expectancy in SSA is now 47 years, an average of 15 years lower than it would be without HIV/AIDS.[158] In addition, young people are inheriting debts and are forced to increase cultivation in order to try to feed more dependents without much knowledge of agricultural techniques, indigenous knowledge, and biodiversity and without much chance of accessing credit and knowledge through community or state institutions.[159] The loss of indigenous knowledge and biodiversity is critical, since these are major assets which become even more important as other tangible resources diminish within affected rural communities.[160]

All of the above factors have resulted in a decline in production. For example, a study conducted in Zimbabwe found that output on smallholder farms decreased by 29% for cattle, 49% for vegetables and 61% for maize for households which had experienced an AIDS-related death.[161] Altogether, maize production had dropped 54%.[162] Cassava production has steadily increased over a five year period and replaced more labour-intensive crops such as maize in an attempt to compensate for lost labour through HIV/AIDS in Malawi, Mozambique, Zambia and Zimbabwe.[163] Foods which are easier to cultivate are often poorer nutritionally and many households also resort to skipping meals. In addition, households suffer loss of livestock as they are used for sources of food during funerals of relatives who have died from HIV/AIDS.[164]

Illness or death has an immediate impact on households. In western Kenya, Onyango et al. found that death-affected households spent an average of $462 per year, compared with $199 for illness-affected households and $21 for non-affected households. With this amount of cash tied up in illness and death, households were less able to invest in agricultural inputs: illness-affected and death-affected households spent 56% and 61% respectively of the amount spent by non-affected households on agricultural inputs.[165]

In considering the likely consequences of HIV/AIDS on the agricultural sector of the hardest hit countries in SEA, Jayne et al. predict that AIDS-related labour shortages may induce labour migration from the urban informal sector into agriculture. They also suggest that for poorer, smallholder households, land will remain a key constraint on income growth. For highly afflicted rural communities, AIDS-induced decapitalization in the form of loss of savings, cattle assets, draft equipment and other assets may become the greatest limits on rural productivity and livelihoods for these communities.[166]

Human capital is depleted, resources are diverted away from agriculture and there is a loss of both farm and non-farm income. There are also the psychosocial impacts of witnessing the illness and death of spouses and parents and of facing possible destitution.[167] When these factors combine, the lack of food and lack of access to food intensify. De Waal terms this the 'new variant famine' since it targets productive adults and more women than men rather than children and the elderly who are the traditional victims of famines.[168] Within communities, women and girls assume care-giving roles which takes time away from productive tasks. Women are the most vulnerable to HIV/AIDS infection and also to the economic impact of HIV/AIDS.[169] Younger girls are also highly susceptible and may be forced to leave school and assume care-giving roles and eventual care of younger siblings as parents die. All of this impacts upon the long-term development potential of women and girls.[170] In Zimbabwe, Senefeld and Polsky found that households with chronically ill adults were more likely to have their children drop out of school and more likely to resort to migration strategies in order to 'cope'.[171] The Southern African Regional Poverty Network (SARPN) asserts that the cycle of poverty and AIDS entrenches a system of chronic impoverishment: "[T]his weakened social fabric means that families cannot recover previous levels of social functioning, and may even resort to strategies that imperil them further, because the negative consequences of such remedies are not immediately apparent".[172]

Figures 2 and 3 below portray scenarios with vulnerable and less vulnerable rural households, both of which experience the migrant male household head returning from an urban area with HIV. Both households eventually experience the death of the male household head. However, for the more vulnerable household, this precipitates a downward spiral which ends with loss of the homestead, homelessness, destitution and the eventual breakup of the household unit. There, the male migrant had been the main cash earner and physical capital is lost as the household head weakens and dies. Through this process, savings have been used and precious assets sold off to pay for medical expenses, costs of care-giving and a funeral. With less cash and less time to farm, the family plants cassava rather than maize. This reduces the need for labour but is a less nutritious source of food, which exacerbates malnutrition and poor health. When the household is forced to sell off livestock, it is unable to recover its herd and thus its assets are diminished. This eliminates another source of protein as well. The household in Figure 2 is more vulnerable since it is unable to diversify sources of farm and non-farm income. In addition, dependency ratios increase with AIDS orphans joining the already struggling household. In a meta-analysis of national nutrition and health surveys in SSA over the past five years, households with more than one orphan were 3.2 times more likely to have claimed food insecurity and hunger than households with only one orphan or no orphans at all.[173]

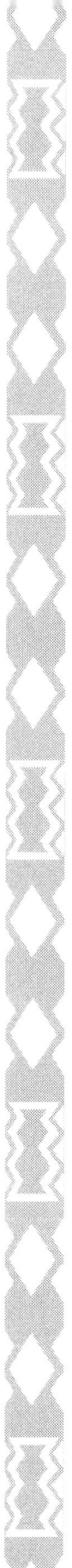

The widow may also be weakened if she contracts HIV or AIDS from her husband. The household's situation is further exacerbated by insecurity of tenure. The youth will attempt to farm, but without the training and knowledge of farming techniques, traditional methods and biodiversity knowledge which normally would be passed on by their parents. Social capital is lost without serious intervention. All of this leads to food insecurity, malnutrition and poor health. At some point, the widow or her daughters may be forced into risky survival strategies just to provide food for the household, further perpetuating the HIV/AIDS cycle. If the household loses the homestead, they are propelled into destitution and are forced to seek out work and shelter; this situation would likely lead to the disintegration of the household. Gillespie maintains that land acquisition by better-off households will likely increase as widows and orphans fail to keep access and/or ownership rights to land after the husband/father dies and may thus lose the chance to rent out the land as another source of income. "The AIDS epidemic is thus intertwined with the way in which power, authority, value and opportunity are distributed within societies."[174]

Figure 2: Vulnerable Rural Household

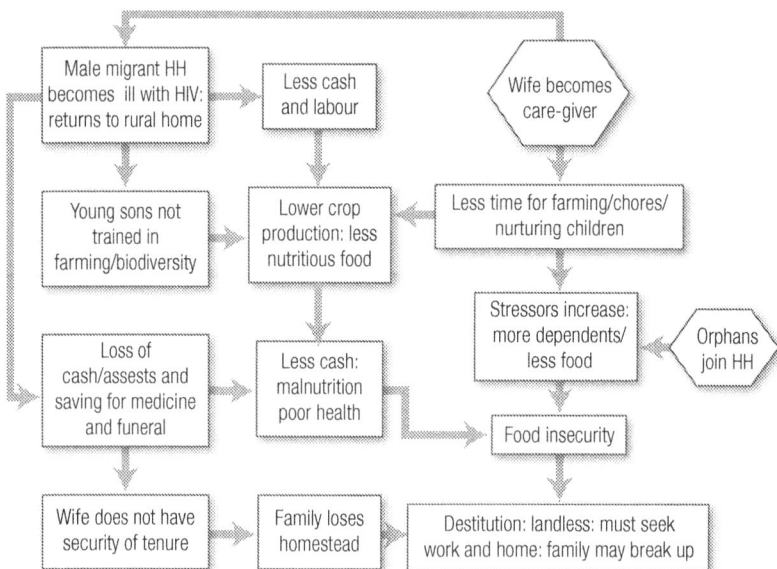

The less vulnerable household in Figure 3 is able to increase off-farm production and to access remittances from two urban migrants. This helps the household to maintain crop production, proper nutrition and food security.

Here also, a female relative migrates to help the household with chores and children. Even though orphans join the household, the burden of care is shared and there is enough food to avoid insecurity. In this situation, security of tenure also ensures household and food security and thus risky survival strategies can be avoided. The two urban migrants would also be able to benefit from food remittances from the household.

Figure 3: More Diversified and Less Vulnerable Rural Household

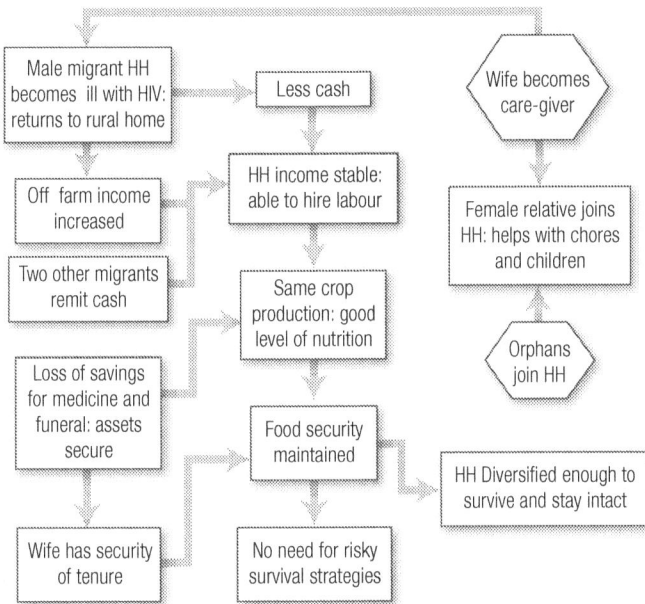

As noted in previous sections, rural and urban households are inexorably intertwined socially and economically. When HIV/AIDS affects households in either or both locales, food and livelihood security is compromised. HIV increases vulnerability to food insecurity, which increases vulnerability to HIV infection and thus HIV can be seen as a shock to household security.[175] Gillespie et al. describe HIV as a 'unique, slow-moving and devastating shock.'[176] When households are stripped of livelihood assets, Mdladla et al. term this a 'creeping emergency' which progressively diminishes the lives and livelihoods of affected households.[177]

Research on the impact of HIV/AIDS on households in Malawi, Zambia and Zimbabwe reveals that HIV-related morbidity and mortality increases vulnerability to food insecurity and causes earlier engagement in distress strategies in response to food insecurity, particularly on the part of poor households.[178] Even though HIV/AIDS affected households might temporarily avoid destitution through various response strategies, in the end they may not be able to avoid a long-term downward spiral in food security and may never recover from the shock.[179] Compared with strategies adopted by other households facing other shocks, the cumulative effect on households impacted by HIV/AIDS may be permanent since these coping strategies are more likely to be irreversible.[180] For example, following a shock to household income, households in Malawi affected by HIV/AIDS took up to 18 months to stabilize, with a new equilibrium income that was about half the pre-shock income levels.[181] As HIV infection rates increase, more households could be food secure on a permanent basis, leading to increased malnutrition. This not only threatens the resilience of food insecure households, but reduced ability to respond may hasten the onset of famine conditions.[182]

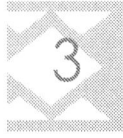

3 DIRECTIONS AND PRIORITIES

3.1 Conceptualizing the Links between Migration, HIV/AIDS and Urban Food Security

As established above, the social and economic relationship between rural and urban areas is symbiotic, and food transfers to urban migrants can exceed urban cash remittances, although remittances remain crucial to rural production. However, HIV/AIDS is undermining and weakening physical and social capital in both rural and urban areas, particularly amongst poorer households. Although migration is a key element of the new social economy, it is also a significant vector of HIV/AIDS.

The linkages between migration, food security and HIV/AIDS constitute a complex web of causal connections and feedback mechanisms. For example, HIV/AIDS is a disease that demonstrably impacts rural food production. Not only does this compromise the food security of rural producers, it could reduce the flow of food from countryside to town (thus making the urban-based migrant more vulnerable to food insecurity). At the same time, the rural household becomes more dependent on cash earnings and remittances for survival, increasing the pressure for remittances. New forms of return "distress" migration to rural areas, simultaneously increasing the burden of provision on the rural household. Again, if the migrant is expected or forced to remit a greater proportion of his or her urban pay packet to compensate for declining agricultural production, their own ability to purchase food may be reduced. Given that migrants spend a large proportion of their wages on necessities such as food, their own diet could suffer. Migrants with HIV/AIDS themselves are, over time and in the absence of ART, likely to be less able to work to full capacity and to remit. The problem here is that migrants are, by most accounts, more vulnerable to HIV infection.

In the absence of definitive research, one way of conceptualizing the links between migration, rural/urban food security and HIV/AIDS is through a more systematic modeling of the potential connections and feedback loops. Figure 4, for example, suggests a set of connections between poverty, urbanization, food insecurity, risky survival strategies and HIV/AIDS. This model is a useful programmatic statement of the potential linkages in the urban setting. However, it does not systematically integrate the rural end of the migration spectrum which, as this paper has argued, is also essential to understanding urban food security.

Figure 4: Links Between Urban Food Insecurity and HIV/AIDS

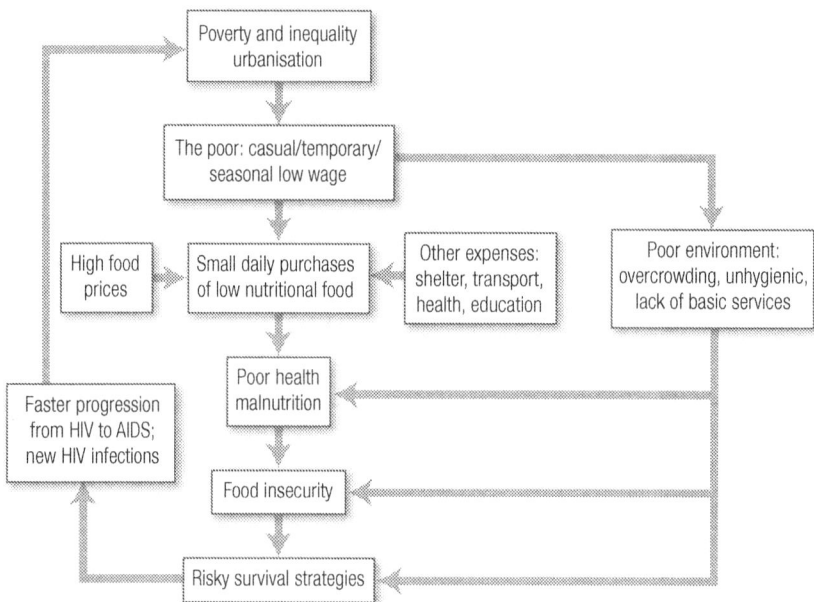

For the poor urban migrant in a cash intensive environment, HIV/AIDS will also potentially propel them into a downward spiral. As Figure 5 shows, with physical capital loss, the migrant will lose capacity to work for cash, which means they will increasingly be unable to meet basic needs, including food. More than likely, food consumption will be the first item to be reduced as cash and savings diminish. The ability of the migrant to engage in urban agriculture will be limited due to their loss of energy and poor health. With less cash for survival, the migrant will be forced to stop remitting altogether or to reduce amounts sent to the rural extended family, placing that family at risk with respect to cash needed for agricultural input and basic needs. If food transfers from the rural family have been reduced, or if food has inferior nutritional quality, the migrant will have less access to nutritious food just when their body needs decent nutrition. These conditions will exacerbate conditions of malnutrition and poor health and will lead to food insecurity.

Figure 5: Linkages between HIV/AIDS, Migration and Food Security

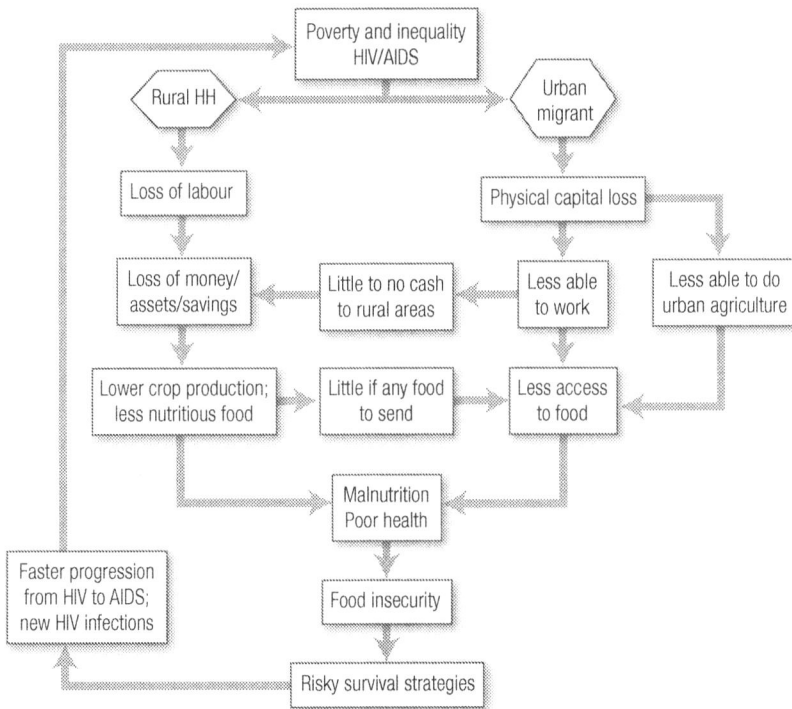

The urban household would be forced to use up savings, sell valuable assets, or borrow money at high interest rates. Dependency would increase on rural and urban based extended family members, without the ability to reciprocate. In the context of food insecurity and deprivation, household members would be highly likely to engage in risky survival strategies, further exacerbating the HIV/AIDS cycle. As the migrant is further debilitated from HIV/AIDS, they will be forced to leave the city and return home to the rural areas for continuous care. This places a further burden on the rural household, not only with respect to burden of care and the required use of assets, but also with loss of urban remittances for agricultural production. If the rural household is vulnerable, this could start a downward cycle resulting in increased participation in risky survival strategies, perpetuation of the HIV/AIDS cycle, and ultimate destitution.

The new social economy which is underpinned by migration will be seriously compromised unless appropriate interventions – driven by praxis oriented research and policy – can be undertaken within the framework of rural and urban food production and access to food to break the vicious cycle of HIV/AIDS, migration and food insecurity. The balance between cash remittances from urban migrants and food transfers from rural households is a delicate one for impoverished, vulnerable households. Thus, if urban migrants are able to access food without compromising other basic needs, this would improve the health of the migrant as well as reinforce the balance between cash remittances for rural production and survival and food transfers to the urban migrant.

3.2   Towards a Synthesis

This publication has highlighted the high urbanization rates and increasing rural-urban linkages in the region, both domestic and cross-border, and demonstrated that rural and urban food security is highly interdependent. It has been further argued that HIV/AIDS has a direct negative impact on urban food security, most notably through the consequent reduction in physical capital and production of food in rural areas and increased burden of dependence of HIV-positive individuals on both urban and rural social units. This precipitates a deepening of poverty at the household level. Yet the three-way linkage between migration, HIV/AIDS and urban food security has yet to be fully researched and understood.

Within this context, there is a need for research-informed interventions to improve the conditions for poor households to create greater food security opportunities and to mitigate the negative impacts of HIV/AIDS on the sustainability of livelihoods in urban centres in Southern and Eastern Africa. However, as the knowledge gaps articulated below make clear, there are contextual variations across the region, and it should be expected that this heterogeneous geography will be reflected in the research outcomes. Developing typologies will therefore be central to the ability of research to contribute meaningfully to the growing need for greater support to poor households and to scale up

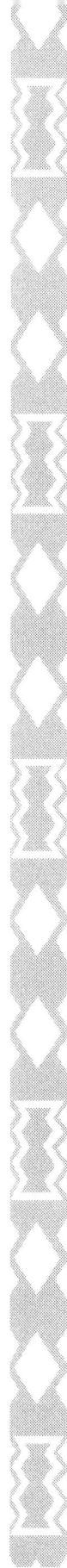

interventions by understanding contextual needs and allowing intervention replication to take place. By so doing, not only is the potential impact of research region-wide, but the outcomes may be useful as international public goods for adaptation to other contexts in which the triple threat of migration, HIV/AIDS and food insecurity is playing itself out (for example, in India).

Emerging from the review, it is possible to identify at least four key knowledge gaps in relation to the three interrelated elements of migration, HIV/AIDS and urban food security within SEA, as follows:

a) Typologies of Reciprocity: Different patterns and systems of urban-rural linkages (migration) at the household level and the economic and nutritional impacts on household food security (quantifying the dimensions of the new social economy of migration).

b) Typologies of Risk: Different patterns and systems of urban-rural linkages (migration) at the household level and the differentiated impacts of HIV and AIDS on household food security (effects on resistance, susceptibility and resilience of households to HIV and AIDS).

c) Typologies of Coping: Impacts of HIV and AIDS on household food security strategies within the context of urban-rural linkages (changes, diversification strategies and the role of migration).

d) Typologies of Intervention: Design of appropriate and supportive policy and programming interventions to address the development challenges posed by the triple threat of migration, HIV/AIDS and food insecurity.

The general research question can be stated as follows:

How does the mobility of people and urban-rural linkages affect the spread of HIV and the impacts of AIDS on food and nutrition security?

Within the broad aim of addressing this question and documenting similarities and differences between contexts within the region, the following research questions provide a starting point for understanding the interactions between migration, HIV/AIDS and food and nutrition security:

a) What is the contribution of rural food production at the household level to the food budget of urban households?

b) To what extent is HIV/AIDS impacting both rural and urban household food security?

c) How and to what degree are these impacts magnified or ameliorated by rural-urban migration and rural-urban linkages at the household level?

d) What role does urban agriculture play, together with other coping strategies, in meeting the food gap of urban households, and is this influenced by HIV and AIDS?

e) Based on the research findings, what policy and programming interventions are required to address the development challenges posed by the triple threat of migration, HIV/AIDS and food insecurity?

Endnotes

1 W. Pendleton et al, *Migration, Remittances and Development in Southern Africa*. SAMP Migration Policy Series No. 44, Cape Town, 2006.

2 J. Crush, B. Williams, E. Gouws and M. Lurie, "Migration and HIV/AIDS in South Africa" *Development Southern Africa* 22 (2005): 293-318; J. Crush, M. Lurie, B. Williams, S. Peberdy, B. Dodson, C. Akileswaran, N. Ansell, M. Gyimah, A. Johnson and B. Rijks, *HIV/AIDS, Population Mobility and Migration in Southern Africa: Defining a Research and Policy Agenda* (Pretoria: IOM, 2005); M. Lurie, "The Epidemiology of Migration and HIV/AIDS in South Africa" *Journal of Ethnic and Migration Studies* 32 (2006): 649-66.

3 Crush et al, *HIV/AIDS, Migration and Population Mobility*.

4 B. Frayne, *Survival of the Poorest: Migration and Food Security in Namibia*, PhD thesis (Kingston: Queen's University, 2001).

5 UN-HABITAT, *State of the World's Cities: Trends in Sub-Saharan Africa* (Nairobi: UN-HABITAT, 2004-2005).

6 UN-HABITAT, *Basic Facts on Urbanization* (New York: UN-HABITAT, 1999).

7 UN-HABITAT, *State of the World's Cities*.

8 C. Kessides, *The Urban Transition in Sub-Saharan Africa: Implications for Economic Growth and Poverty Reduction* (Washington: The World Bank, 2005).

9 F. Ellis and N. Harris, "New Thinking About Urban and Rural Development" (Keynote Paper for DFID Sustainable Development Retreat, University of Surrey, Guildford, 2004).

10 J. Gugler, "The Son of the Hawk Does Not Remain Abroad: The Urban-Rural Connection in Africa" *African Studies Review* 45 (2002): 35.

11 Ibid, p. 137.

12 D. Potts, "Urban Unemployment and Migrants in Africa: Evidence from Harare 1985-1994" *Development and Change* 31 (2000): 879-910.

13 J. Andersson, "Reinterpreting the Rural–Urban Connection: Migration Practices and Socio-Cultural Dispositions of Buhera Workers in Harare" *Africa* 71 (2001): 82-112.

14 H. Englund, "The Village in the City, the City in the Village: Migrants in Lilongwe" *Journal of Southern African Studies* 28 (2002): 137-154.

15 C. Cross, T. Mngadi and T. Mbhele, "Constructing Migration: Infrastructure, Poverty and

Development in KwaZulu-Natal" *Development Southern Africa* 15 (1998): 635-59.

16   C. Tacoli, "Rural–Urban Interactions: A Guide to the Literature" *Environment and Urbanization* 10 (1998): 147-66.

17   S. Owuor, "Urban households ruralizing their livelihoods: The changing nature of urban-rural linkages in an East African town." Paper presented at the African Studies Centre Seminar Series, Leiden, December 2004.

18   W. Smit, "The Rural Linkages of Urban Households in Durban, South Africa" *Environment and Urbanization* 10 (1998): 77-87.

19   Cross et al, "Constructing Migration."

20   Frayne, B. and W. Pendleton. "Migration in Namibia: Combining Macro and Micro Approaches to Research Design and Analysis" *International Migration Review* 35(4) (2001): 1054-1085.

21   A. Spiegel, V. Watson, and P. Wilkinson. 1996. Domestic Diversity and Fluidity in Some African Households in greater Cape Town. *Social Dynamics* 22 (1): 7-30.

22   J. Crush, S. Peberdy and V. Williams, "International Migration in Southern Africa" Report for Global Commission on International Migration, Geneva, 2005.

23   S. Chant, *Gender and Migration in Developing Countries* (London: Belhaven Press, 1992).

24   C. Gadio and C. Rakowski, "Survival or Empowerment? Crisis and Temporary Migration Among the Serer Millet pounders of Senegal" *Women's Studies International Forum* 18 (1995): 431-43.

25   Tacoli, "Rural–Urban Interactions."

26   Statistics South Africa, *Migration and Changing Settlement Patterns: Multilevel Data for Policy* (Pretoria: Statistics South Africa, 2006).

27   Ibid.

28   Statistics South Africa, *Migration and Urbanization in South Africa* (Pretoria: Statistics South Africa, 2006).

29   W. Pendleton, D. LeBeau and C. Tapscott, "Socio-Economic Study of the Ondangwa/Oshakati Nexus Area" Research Report. Namibian Institute for Social and Economic Research. (Windhoek: University of Namibia, 1992); A. Pomuti and I. Tvedten, "Namibia: Urbanization in the 1990s" In Namibian Economic Policy Research Unit Publication No. 6, *In Search of Research* (Windhoek: Nepru, 1998); B. Frayne, and W. Pendleton. *Mobile Namibia: Trends in National and International Migration.* SAMP Migration Policy Series No. 27, Cape Town, 2003; B. Frayne, "Rural Productivity and Urban Survival in Namibia: Eating Away from Home" *Journal of Contemporary African Studies* 23 (2005): 51-76.

30   Kessides, *The Urban Transition.*

31   UN-HABITAT, *State of the World's Cities.*

32   C. Murray, *Families Divided: The Impact of Migrant Labour in Lesotho* (New York: Cambridge University Press, 1981); R. Moorsom, *Underderdevelopment and Labour Migration: The Contract Labour System in Namibia* (Bergen, Norway: Christian Michelsen Institute, 1995); D. Potts and C. Mutambirwa, "'Basics Are Now a Luxury': Perceptions of Structural Adjustment's

Impact on Rural and Urban Areas in Zimbabwe" *Environment and Urbanization* 10 (1998): 55-76.

33   A. Marsh and M. Seely, eds., *Oshanas. Sustaining People, Environment and Development in Central Owambo, Namibia* (Windhoek: DRFN and SIDA, 1992); C. Rogerson, "Forgotten Places, Abandoned Places: Migration Research Issues in South Africa" In J. Baker and T. Aina, eds., *The Migration Experience in Africa* (Uppsala: Nordiska Afrikainstitutet, 1995); D. McDonald, "Lest the Rhetoric Begin: Migration, Population and the Environment in Southern Africa" *Geoforum* 30 (1999): 13-25.

34   H. Evans and G. Pirzada, "Rural Households as Producers" in Baker and Aina, *The Migration Experience*, pp. 65-83; S. Devereux and T. Naeraa, "Drought and Survival in Rural Namibia" *Journal of Southern African Studies* 22 (1996): 421-40.

35   B. Frayne, "Migration and Urban Survival Strategies in Windhoek, Namibia" *Geoforum* 35 (2004): 489-505.

36   J. Crush and D. McDonald, eds., *Transnationalism and New African Immigration to South Africa* (Cape Town and Toronto: SAMP and CAAS, 2002).

37   B. Dodson, *Women on the Move: Gender and Cross-Border Migration to South Africa*. SAMP Migration Policy Series No. 9, Cape Town, 1998.

38   Evans and Pirzada, "Rural Households as Producers."

39   J. Crush, *Covert Operations: Clandestine Migration, Temporary work, and Immigration Policy in South Africa*. SAMP Migration Policy Series No. 1, Cape Town, 1997.

40   McDonald, *On Borders*, p. 232.

41   J. Crush and W. James, eds. *Crossing Boundaries* (Cape Town and Ottawa: Idasa and IDRC, 1995).

42   This paper uses the term "irregular migration" recently proposed by the Global Commission on International Migration.

43   J. Crush, "The Discourse and Dimensions of Irregularity in Post-Apartheid South Africa" *International Migration* 37 (1999): 125-51.

44   C. Rogerson, *Building Skills: Cross-Border Migrants and the South African Construction Industry*. SAMP Migration Policy Series No. 11, Cape Town, 1999; J. Crush, C. Mather, F. Mathebula and D. Lincoln, *Borderline Farming: Foreign Migrants in South African Commercial Agriculture*. SAMP Migration Policy Series No. 16, Cape Town, 2000.

45   McDonald, *On Borders*.

46   Dodson, *Women on the Move*.

47   B. Dodson, "Women on the Move: Gender and Cross border Migration to South Africa from Lesotho, Mozambique and Zimbabwe" In D. McDonald, ed., *On Borders*, pp. 119-50; K. Datta, "Gender, Labour Markets and Female Migration in and from Botswana" In D. Simon, ed., *South Africa in Southern Africa: Reconfiguring the Region* (Oxford: James Currey, 1998), pp. 206-21.

48   Dodson, "Women on the Move," p. 124.

49   Ibid; B. Dodson, "Discrimination by Default? Gender Concerns in South African Immigration Policy" *Africa Today* 48 (2001): 72-89.

50   Dodson, "Women on the Move," p. 126.

51   S. Peberdy and C. Rogerson, "Transnationalism and Non-South African Entrepreneurs in South Africa's Small, Medium and Micro-enterprise (SMME) Economy" *Canadian Journal of African Studies* 34 (2000): 20-40.

52   S. Peberdy and C. Rogerson, "Creating New Spaces? Immigrant Entrepreneurship in South Africa's SMME Economy" In R. Kloosterman and J. Rath, eds., *Immigrant Entrepreneurs: Venturing Abroad in the Age of Globalization* (Oxford: Berg, 2003); S. Peberdy and J. Crush, "Invisible Travellers, Invisible Trade? Informal Sector Cross Border Trade and the Maputo Corridor Spatial Development Initiative" *South African Geographical Journal* 83 (2001): 115-23; S. Peberdy, "Mobile Entrepreneurship: Informal Cross-Border Trade and Street Trade in South Africa" *Development Southern Africa* 17 (2000): 201-19; S. Peberdy, "Border Crossings: Small Entrepreneurs and Informal Sector Cross Border Trade Between South Africa and Mozambique" *Tjidschrift voor Economische en Sociale Geographie* 91 (2000): 361-78; V. Muzvidziwa, "Cross-Border Trade: A Strategy for Climbing Out of Poverty in Masvingo, Zimbabwe" *Zambezia* 25 (1998): 29-58; J. Macamo, *Estimates of Unrecorded Cross-Border Trade between Mozambique and Her Neighbors: Implications for Food Security (Final Report).* Unpublished paper for the Regional Economic Development Support Office for Eastern and Southern Africa, USAID, 1998; I. Minde and T. Nakhumwa, *Informal Cross-Border Trade Between Malawi and Her Neighbouring Countries.* Unpublished paper for the Regional Economic evelopment Support Office for Eastern and Southern Africa, USAID, 1997.

53   S. Peberdy and J. Oucho, "Migration and Poverty" Unpublished paper for the ACP-EU Parliamentary Committee, Cape Town, 2002; S. Parnell and D. Wooldridge, eds., "Social Capital and Social Inclusion in the City of Johannesburg and the Implications for Urban Government" Unpublished report for the City of Johannesburg, 2001.

54   B. Frayne, "Migrants, Remittances and the Southern African Economy: Terms of Reference" Unpublished paper for the Southern African Migration Project, 2002.

55   J. Iliffe, *The African AIDS Epidemic: A History* (London: James Currey, 2006); S. Gillespie, "AIDS, Poverty and Hunger: An Overview" In S. Gillespie, ed., *AIDS, Poverty and Hunger: Challenges and Responses. Highlights of the International Conference on HIV/AIDS and Food and Nutrition Security, Durban, South Africa, 14-16 April, 2005* (2006).

56   T. Barnett and D. Topouzis, *FAO and HIV/AIDS, Towards a Food and Livelihoods Security Based Strategic Response* (Rome: FAO, 2003).

57   UNAIDS, *AIDS Epidemic Update* (Geneva: UNAIDS and WHO, 2005).

58   UNDP, *Human Development Report Documents Catastrophic Impact of AIDS in Africa* (New York: UNDP, 2004).

59   UNAIDS/WHO, *Progess on Global Access.*

60   UNAIDS, *AIDS Epidemic Update.*

61   E. Gomo, Z. Jokomo, R. Mate and J. Chipika, *Zimbabwe Human Development Report 2003: Redirecting Our Responses to HIV/AIDS* (Harare: Institute of Development Studies, University of Zimbabwe, 2003).

62 City of Bulawayo, *Annual Report of the Director of Health Services* (Bulawayo: City of Bulawayo, 2000).

63 Gomo et al, *Zimbabwe Human Development Report 2003.*

64 A. Tibaijuka, *Report of the Fact-Finding Mission to Zimbabwe to Assess the Scope and Impact of Operation Murambatsvina* (New York: United Nations, 2005).

65 Human Rights Watch, *Clear the Filth: Mass Evictions and Demolitions in Zimbabwe.* Briefing Paper, (New York: Human Rights Watch, 2005).

66 Department of Health, South Africa, *National HIV and Syphilis Antenatal Sero-Prevalence Survey in South Africa, 2004* (Pretoria: Department of Health, 2005).

67 UNAIDS, *AIDS Epidemic Update.*

68 R. Cockett, "Chasing the Rainbow: A Survey of South Africa" *The Economist* April 8, 2006: 1-12.

69 Ministry of Health and Social Welfare, Swaziland, *9th Round of National HIV Serosurveillance in Women Attending Antenatal Care at Health Facilities in Swaziland: Survey Report* (Mbabane, Ministry of Health and Social Welfare Swaziland, 2005).

70 Ministry of Health and Social Welfare Lesotho, 2005 as cited in UNAIDS, *AIDS Epidemic Update.*

71 UNAIDS, *AIDS Epidemic Update.*

72 Ministry of Health and Population Malawi, *HIV Sentinel Surveillance Report 2003* (Lilongwe: Ministry of Health and Population, 2003).

73 UNAIDS, *AIDS Epidemic Update.*

74 Ibid.

75 National HIV/AIDS Council Zambia, *ANC Sentinel Surveillance of HIV/AIDS Trends in Zambia, 1994-2002* (Lusaka: Tropical Diseases Research Center, 2002).

76 Grupo tematico VIH/SIDA Angola, "A luta e epidemia de VIH/SIDA como uma priordade nacional" Presentacao 11 Dezembro (Luanda: Ministerio de saude do Angola, UNAIDS, 2002) cited in UNAIDS, *AIDS Epidemic Update.*

77 UNAIDS, AIDS Epidemic Update.

78 Ibid.

79 Ministry of Health, Uganda, *STD/HIV/AIDS Surveillance Report* (Kampala: Ministry of Health, 2003).

80 Gender Issues in HIV/AIDS and Food/Nutrition security among Internally Displaced People's Camps in Uganda. RENEWAL study (ongoing), Makerere University.

81 UNAIDS, *AIDS Epidemic Update.*

82 M. Wagah, *Background Paper on HIV/AIDS, Food and Nutrition Security in Kenya.* RENEWAL, International Food Policy & Research Institute, Washington, D.C., 2005.

83 E. Kissling, E. Allison, J. Seeley, S. Russell, M. Bachmann, S. Musgrave, and S. Heck,

"Fisherfolk are Among Groups Most at Risk of HIV: Cross-country Analysis of Prevalence and Numbers Infected" *AIDS* 19 (2005): 1939-46.

84   S. Nko et al., "Secretive Females or Swaggering males? An Assessment of the Quality of Sexual Partnership Reporting in Rural Tanzania" *Social Science and Medicine* 59 (2004): 299-310.

85   UNAIDS, *AIDS Epidemic Update*; Central Intelligence Agency (CIA), *The World Factbook* (Washington: CIA, 2005).

86   Federal Ministry of Health Ethiopia, *AIDS in Ethiopia: 5th Report* (Addis Ababa: Federal Ministry of Health, Disease Prevention and Control Department, 2004).

87   S. Lautzke et al. "Risk and Vulnerability in Ethiopia: Learning from the Past, Responding to the Present, Preparing for the Future." Report for the US Agency for International Development (USAID), Feinstein International Famine Centre and Inter-University Initiative on Humanitarian Studies and Field Practice, 2003.

88   Federal Ministry of Health Ethiopia, *AIDS in Ethiopia*; UNAIDS/WHO, *Progress on Global Access to HIV Antiretroviral Therapy: An Update on '3 by 5'* (Geneva: UNAIDS/WHO, 2005); UNAIDS, *2004 Report on the Global AIDS Epidemic* (Geneva: UNAIDS, 2004).

89   S. Drimie, B. Frayne and G. Tafesse, *Ethiopia Background Paper: HIV/AIDS, Food and Nutrition Security*. RENEWAL, International Food Policy & Research Institute, Washington, D.C., 2005.

90   WHO, *The 2004 First National Second Generation HIV/AIDS/STI Sentinel Surveillance Survey Among Antenatal Care Women Attending Maternity and Child Care Clinics, Tuberculosis and STD Patients* (Somalia: WHO, 2005).

91   M. Jooma, "Southern Africa Assessment: Food Security and HIV/AIDS" *Africa Security Review* 14 (2005): 59-66.

92   World Bank, *Poverty and Hunger: Issues and Options for Food Security in Developing Countries* (Washington: World Bank, 1986); D. Maxwell, "The Political Economy of Urban Food Security in Sub-Saharan Africa" *World Development* 27 (1999): 1939-53.

93   S. Maxwell, "Food Security: A Post-modern Perspective" *Food Policy* 21 (1996): 155-70; S. Hendriks, "The Challenges Facing Empirical Estimation of Household Food (In)security in South Africa" *Development Southern Africa* 22 (2005): 103-23.

94   C. Barrett, "Does Food Aid Stabilize Food Availability?" *Economic Development and Cultural Change* 49 (2001): 335-49.

95   S. Devereux and S. Maxwell, "Introduction" In S. Devereux and S. Maxwell, eds., *Food Security in Sub Saharan Africa* (Pietermaritzburg: University of Natal Press, 2001), pp. 1-12.

96   E. Dowler, "Food and Poverty: Insights from the 'North'," *Development Policy Review* 21 (2003): 569-614.

97   Hendriks, "Challenges."

98   Jooma, "Southern Africa Assessment."

99   C. Becker, A. Jamer and A. Morrison, *Beyond Urban Bias in Africa* (Portsmouth, NH:

Heinemann, 1994); R. Stren, R. White and J. Whitney, *Sustainable Cities: Urbanization and the Environment in International Perspective* (Boulder, CO: Westview, 1992).

100   UNCHS, *An Urbanizing World: Global Report on Human Settlements, 1996* (Oxford: Oxford University Press, 1996).

101   A. de Haan, "Urban Poverty and Its Alleviation: Introduction" *IDS Bulletin* 28 (1997): 1-8; UNCHS, *An Urbanizing World.*

102   C. Rakodi, "A Livelihoods Approach – Conceptual Issues and Definitions" In C. Rakodi with T. Lloyd-Jones, eds., *Urban Livelihoods: A People-centred Approach to Reducing Poverty*, (London: Earthscan, 2002), pp. 3-22; D. Mitlin, "Understanding Chronic Poverty in Urban Areas" *International Planning Studies* 10 (2005): 3-19.

103   L. Kironde, "Access to Land by the Urban Poor in Tanzania: Some Findings from Dar es Salaam" *Environment and Urbanization* 7 (1995): 77-96.

104   D. Maxwell, C. Levin, M. Armar-Klemesu, M. Ruel, S. Morris and C. Ahiadeke, *Urban Livelihoods and Food and Nutrition Security in Greater Accra, Ghana* IFPRI Research Report 112 (Washington: IFPRI, 2000); J. Garrett and M. Ruel, "Food and Nutrition in an Urbanizing World" *Choices: The Magazine of Food, Farm and Resource Issues* 14 (1999); J. Pryer, S. Roger and A. Rahman, "Work-disabling Illness as a Shock for Livelihoods and Poverty in Dhaka Slums, Bangladesh" *International Planning Studies* 10 (2005): 69-80.

105   Maxwell, "The Political Economy of Urban Food Security."

106   Garrett and Ruel, "Food and Nutrition."

107   M. Chopra, "Equity Issues in HIV/AIDS, Nutrition and Food Security in Southern Africa" Regional Network for Equity in Health in Southern Africa, Equinet Discussion Paper 11, 2003.

108   S. Basta, M. Soekirman, D. Karyadi and N. Scrimshaw, "Iron Deficiency Anemia and the Productivity of Adult Males in Indoensia" *American Journal of Clinical Nutrition* 32 (1979): 916-25.

109   Garrett and Ruel, "Food and Nutrition."

110   Chopra, "Equity Issues in HIV/AIDS."

111   Ibid.

112   de Haan, "Urban Poverty and Its Alleviation"; M. Ruel et al, *Urban Challenges to Nutrition Security: A Review of Food Security, Health and Care in Cities*, Food Consumption and Nutrition Division Discussion Paper No. 51 (Washington: IFPRI, 1998); P. Amis, "Making Sense of Urban Poverty" *Environment and Urbanization* 7 (1995): 145-57; C. Moser, "Urban Social Policy and Poverty Reduction" *Environment and Urbanization* 7 (1995): 159-71.

113   Frayne, "Rural Productivity and Urban Survival."

114   Frayne, *Survival of the Poorest.*

115   D. Potts, "Worker-peasants and Farmer-housewives in Africa: The Debate About 'Committed' Farmers, Access to Land and Agricultural Production" *Journal of Southern African Studies* 26 (2000): 807-32; L. Bijlmakers, M. Basset and D. Sanders, *Health and Structural Adjustment in Rural and Urban Zimbabwe*, Research Report No. 101 (Uppsala: Nordiska Afrikainstitutet,

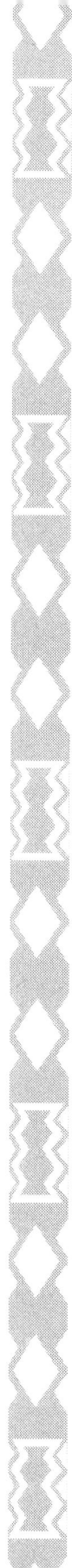

1996); Potts and Mutambirwa, "'Basics Are Now a Luxury."

116   J. Oucho, *Urban Migrants and Rural Development in Kenya* (Nairobi, 1996), p. 147.

117   This section is based on B. Dodson and J. Crush, "Mobile Deathlihoods: Migration and HIV/ AIDS in Africa," Report for UNAIDS, 2003.

118   M. Haour-Knipe and R. Rector, eds., *Crossing Borders: Migration, Ethnicity and AIDS* (London: Taylor & Francis, 1996); J. Caldwell et al, "Mobility, Migration, STDs and AIDS: An Essay on Sub-Saharan Africa" In G. Herdt, ed., *Sexual Cultures and Migration in the Case of AIDS* (Oxford: Clarendon, 1997); J. Decosas and A. Adrien, "Migration and HIV" *AIDS* 11 (Suppl. A) (1997): S77-84; E. Kalipeni, S. Craddock and J. Ghosh, "Mapping the AIDS Pandemic in Eastern and Southern Africa: A Critical Overview" In E. Kalipeni, S. Craddock, J. Oppong and J. Ghosh, eds., *HIV & AIDS in Africa* (Oxford: Blackwell, 2004), pp. 58-69.

119   R. Skeldon, "Population Mobility and HIV/AIDS Mobility in South-East Asia: An Assessment and Analysis" (New York: UNDP, 2000); UN South East Asia HIV and Development Project, *Mobile Populations and HIV Vulnerability: Selected Responses in South East Asia* (New York: UNDP, 2002); D. Simonet, "The AIDS Epidemic and Migrants in South Asia and South-East Asia" *International Migration* 42 (2004): 35-67; Crush et al, *HIV/AIDS, Population Mobility and Migration.*

120   UNDP South East Asia HIV and Development Project, "Land Transport and HIV Vulnerability: A Development Challenge" (Bangkok, 2002); UNDP South East Asia HIV and Development Project, "Building an Alliance with the Transport Sector in HIV Vulnerability Reduction" (Bangkok, 2002); J. Anarfi, "Sexuality, Migration and AIDS in Ghana: A Socio-Behavioural Study" *Health Transition Review* 3 (1993): 45-67; M. Brockerhoff and A. Biddlecom, "Migration, Sexual Behaviour and the Risk of HIV in Kenya" *International Migration Review* 33 (1999): 833-56; J. Crush, T. Ulicki, T. Tseane and E. Jansen Van Vuuren, "Undermining Labour: The Rise of Sub-Contracting in South African Gold Mines" *Journal of Southern African Studies* 27 (2001): 5-32; M. Lurie, "The Epidemiology of Migration and AIDS in South Africa" In R. Cohen, ed., *Migration and Health in Southern Africa* (Cape Town: Van Schaik, 2003), pp. 100-13.

121   G. Ramjee and E. Gouws, "Prevalence of HIV Among Truck Drivers Visiting Sex Workers in KwaZulu-Natal, South Africa" *Sexually Transmitted Diseases* 29 (2002): 44-9; IOM, *HIV and Mobile Workers: A Review of Risks and Programmes among Truckers in West Africa* (Geneva: IOM, 2005).

122   D. Wilson, "Prevention of HIV Infection Through Peer Education and Condom Promotion Among Truck Drivers and their Sexual Partners in Tanzania, 1990-93" *AIDS Care* 12 (2000): 27-40; D. Wilson et al, *Corridors of Hope in Southern Africa: HIV Prevention Needs and Opportunities in Four Border Towns* (Arlington, VA: Family Health International, 2000); D. Wilson et al, *Lesotho and Swaziland: HIV/AIDS Risk Assessment at Cross-Border and Migrant Sites in Southern Africa* (Arlington, VA: Family Health International, 2001).

123   C. Campbell, *Letting Them Die: How HIV/AIDS Prevention Programmes Often Fail* (Oxford: 2003).

124   A. Chapoto and T. Jane, "Socio-economic characteristics of individuals afflicted by AIDS-related prime-age mortality in Zambia" Draft paper prepared for the IFPRI/Renewal Conference on HIV/AIDS and Food and Nutrition Security, Durban South Africa, 14-16 April, 2005.

125 D. Bryceson and J. Fonseca, "A Dying Peasantry? Interactive Impact of Famine and HIV/AIDS in Rural Malawi" Paper presented at the international Conference on HIV/AIDS and Food and Nutrition Security, Durban, 14-16 April, 2005.

126 C. MacPhail, B. Williams and C. Campbell, "Relative Risk of HIV Infection Among Young Men and Women in a South African Township" *International Journal of STD and AIDS* 13 (2002): 331-42.

127 N. Ansell and L. Van Blerk, *HIV/AIDS and Children's Migration in Southern Africa*. SAMP Migration Policy Series No. 33, Cape Town, 2004.

128 R. Skeldon, "Rural–Urban Migration and Its Implications for Poverty Alleviation" *Asia-Pacific Population Journal*, 12 (1997): 3-16.

129 de Haan, "Urban Poverty and Its Alleviation."

130 Tacoli, "Rural–Urban Interactions" p. 151; N. Kanji, *Review of Urbanization Issues Affecting Children and Women in the Eastern and Southern African Region* (New York: UNICEF, 1996), cited in S. Owuor, "Rural Livelihood Sources for Urban Households" African Studies Centre Working Paper 51/2003 (Leiden, Netherlands: African Studies Centre, 2003); C. Tacoli, "The Changing Scale and Nature of Rural–Urban Interactions: Recent Developments and New Agendas" In UNCHS/HABITAT, *Regional Development Planning and Management of Urbanization: Experiences from Developing Countries* (Nairobi: UNCHS/HABITAT, 1997), pp. 150-61.

131 V. Jamal and J. Weeks, "The Vanishing Rural–Urban Gap in Sub-Saharan Africa" *International Labour Review* 127 (1988): p. 288.

132 Frayne, "Rural Productivity and Urban Survival."

133 Owuor, "Rural Livelihood Sources"; Smit, "The Rural Linkages of Urban Households"; D. Foeken and S. Owuor, "Multi-spatial Livelihoods in Sub-Saharan Africa: Rural Farming by Urban Households — The Case of Nakuru Town, Kenya" In M. de Bruijn, R. van Dijk and D. Foeken, eds., *The Rural–Urban Interface in Africa: Expansion and Adaptation* (Uppsala: The Scandinavian Institute of African Studies, 2001), pp. 295-302.

134 J. Baker, "Rural–Urban Links and Economic Differentiation in Northwest Tanzania" *African Rural and Urban Studies* 3 (1996): 25-48.

135 There is a pervasive view in the literature, originating in the underdevelopment paradigm of the 1970s, that migration has always had a very negative impact on levels of rural production and productivity.

136 de Haan, "Urban Poverty and Its Alleviation," p. 29.

137 K. Brock and N. Coulibaly, "Sustainable Livelihoods Project: Mali Country Report" (Sussex: IDS, 1999).

138 S. Findley, "Migration and Family Interactions in Africa" In A. Adepoju, ed., *Family, Population and Development in Africa* (London: Zed Books, 1997), p. 126.

139 Frayne, "Rural Productivity and Urban Survival."

140 C. Tacoli, M. Bah, S. Cisse, B. Diyamett, G. Diallo, F. Lerise, D. Okali, E. Okpara and J. Olawoye, "Changing Rural–Urban Linkages in Mali, Nigeria and Tanzania" *Environment and Urbanization* 15 (2003): 13-23.

141 H. Simelane, "Labour Migration and Rural Transformation in Post-colonial Swaziland" *Journal of Contemporary African Studies* 13 (1995): 207-26.

142 D. Drakakis-Smith, "Strategies for Meeting Basic Food Needs in Harare" In J. Baker and P. Pedersen, eds., *The Rural–Urban Interface in Africa* (Uppsala, 1992).

143 A. S. Fall, "Migrants' Long-distance Relationships and Social Networks in Dakar" *Environment and Urbanization* 10 (1998): 135-45.

144 Owuor, "Rural Livelihood Sources."

145 F. Ellis and J. Sumberg, "Food Production, Urban Areas and Policy Responses" *World Development* 26 (1998): 213-25.

146 D. Maxwell, "Alternative Food Security Strategy: A Household Analysis of Urban Agriculture in Kampala" *World Development* 23 (1995): 1669-81.

147 B. Sanyal, *Urban Cultivation in East Africa: People's Response to Urban Poverty.* (Paris: The Food Energy Nexus Programme, United Nations University, 1986); Jamal and Weeks, "The Vanishing Rural–Urban Gap."

148 D. Freeman, *A City of Farmers: Informal Urban Agriculture in the Open Spaces of Nairobi, Kenya* (Montreal: McGill-Queen's Press, 1991).

149 A. Hovorka, "Entrepreneurial Opportunities in Botswana: (Re)Shaping Urban Agriculture Discourse" *Journal of Contemporary African Studies* 22 (2004): 367-88.

150 D. Freeman, "Survival Strategy or Business Training Ground? The Significance of Urban Agriculture for the Advancement of Women in African Cities" *African Studies Review* 36 (1993): 1-22.

151 B. Mbiba, *Urban Agriculture in Zimbabwe* (Aldershot: Avebury, 1995); M. Mlozi, I. Lupanga and Z. Mvena, "Urban Agriculture as a Survival Strategy in Tanzania" In J. Baker and P. Pedersen, *The Rural–Urban Interface in Africa* (Uppsala, 1992).

152 Chopra, "Equity Issues in HIV/AIDS," p. 14.

153 P. Piot and P. Pinstrup-Andersen, *AIDS: The New Challenge to Food Security.* 2001-2002 IFPRI Annual Report Essay (Washington: IFPRI, 2002).

154 Gillespie, *AIDS, Poverty and Hunger.*

155 UNAIDS/FAO, *Sustainable Agricultural/ Rural Development and Vulnerability to the AIDS Epidemic* (New York: UNAIDS, 1999).

156 FAO, *Mitigating the Impact of HIV/AIDS on Food Security and Rural Poverty* (New York: FAO, 2005).

157 L. Haddad and S. Gillespie, "Effective Food and Nutrition Policy Responses to HIV/AIDS: What We Know and What We Need to Know" *Journal of International Development* 13 (2005): 487-511.

158 Jooma, "Southern Africa Assessment."

159 Chopra, "Equity Issues in HIV/AIDS."

160 Southern African Humanitarian Information Network for a Coordinated Disaster Response

(SAHIMS), "The Impact of HIV/AIDS on Agriculture" (31 January 2005).

161   UNAIDS, *AIDS Epidemic Update December 2002* (Geneva: UNAIDS, 2002).

162   P. Kwaramba, *The Socio-Economic Impact of HIV/AIDS on Communal Agricultural Production Systems in Zimbabwe* (Harare: Zimbabwe Farmers' Union and Friederich Ebert Stiftung, 1997).

163   Jooma, "Southern Africa Assessment."

164   T. Barnett and G. Rugelama, "HIV/AIDS: A Critical Health and Development Issue" In P. Pinstrup-Andersen, ed., *Food and Nutrition Issues in the 21st Century* (Washington: IFPRI, 2001).

165   S. Onyango, B. Swallow and S. Mukoya-Wangia, "Effects of HIV/AIDS-related Illness and Deaths on Agricultural Production in the Nyando Basin of Western Kenya" Paper presented at the International Conference on HIV/AIDS and Food and Nutritional Security, Durban, South Africa, 14-16 April 2005.

166   T. Jayne, M. Villarreal, P. Pingali and G. Hemrich, "HIV/AIDS and the Agricultural Sector in Eastern and Southern Africa: Anticipating the Consequences" Paper presented at the International Conference on HIV/AIDS and Food and Nutritional Security, Durban, South Africa, 14-16 April 2005.

167   G. Mutangara, H. Jackson and D. Mukurazita, eds., *AIDS and the African Smallholder Agriculture* (Harare: Southern African AIDS Information Dissemination Service (SAFAIDS), 1999).

168   Southern African Regional Poverty Network (SARPN), *Does HIV/AIDS Imply 'A New Variant Famine'?* (South Africa: SARPN, 2005).

169   Oxfam-Great Britain, *The Underlying Causes of the Food Crisis in the Southern Africa region – Malawi, Mozambique, Zambia and Zimbabwe* (Oxford: Oxfam Great Britain, 28 January 2005).

170   Jooma, "Southern Africa Assessment."

171   S. Senefeld and K. Polsky, "Chronically Ill Households, Food Security and Coping Strategies in Rural Zimbabwe" Paper presented at the International Conference on HIV/AIDS and Food and Nutritional Security, Durban, South Africa, 14-16 April 2005.

172   SARPN, "Does HIV/AIDS Imply".

173   J. Rivers, J. Mason, E. Silvestre, M. Mahy, R. Monasch and S. Gillespie, "The Nutritional and Food Security Status of Orphans and Vulnerable Children in Sub-Saharan Africa" Paper presented at the International Conference on HIV/AIDS and Food and Nutritional Security, Durban, South Africa, 14-16 April 2005.

174   S. Gillespie, "AIDS, Poverty and Hunger: An Overview" In S. Gillespie, ed., *AIDS, Poverty and Hunger: Challenges and Responses* (Durban, 2006), p.12.

175   S. Gillespie, L. Haddad and R. Jackson, "HIV/AIDS, Food and Nutrition Security: Impacts and Actions," Paper prepared for the 28th Session of the ACC/SCN Symposium on Nutrition and HIV/AIDS (Washington: IFPRI, 2005); C. Baylies, "The Impact of AIDS on Rural Households in Africa: A Shock Like Any Other?" *Development and Change* 33 (2002): 611-32; Southern

African Development Community (SADC), *Towards Identifying the Impact of HIV/AIDS on Food Insecurity in Southern Africa and Implications for Responses: Findings from Malawi, Zambia and Zimbabwe* (Harare: SADC Food, Agriculture and Natural Resources Vulnerability Assessment Committee, 2003); Hendriks, "The Challenges."

176   Gillespie et al, "HIV/AIDS, Food and Nutrition Security."

177   P. Mdladla, N. Marshland, J. Van Zyl and S. Drimie, *Towards Identifying the Vulnerability of HIV/AIDS Affected Households to Food Insecurity. The RVAC-UNAIDS Experience: Challenges and Opportunities*, Draft Technical Note: Measuring the Impact of HIV/AIDS on Food Security (Johannesburg: 9-11 September, 2003).

178   SADC, *Towards Identifying the Impact*.

179   Ibid.

180   Gillespie, "HIV/AIDS, Food and Nutrition Security." S. Kadiyala and S. Gillespie, *Rethinking Food Aid to Fight AIDS*, Food Consumption and Nutrition Division Paper No. 159 (Washington: IFPRI, 2003).

181   W. Masanjala, "HIV/AIDS, Household Expenditure and Consumption Dynamics in Malawi" Paper presented at the International Conference on HIV/AIDS and Food and Nutritional Security, Durban, South Africa, 14-16 April 2005.

182   Gillespie et al, "HIV/AIDS, Food and Nutrition Security."

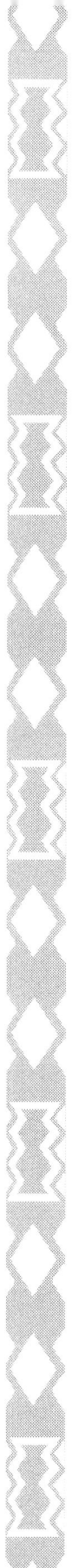

www.ingramcontent.com/pod-product-compliance
Lightning Source LLC
Chambersburg PA
CBHW080850300326

41935CB00042B/1741